Nursing care

in Psychiatry

The Complete Guide

ALEXANDRE CAREWELL

Table of contents

« *Psychiatry is not simply the art of diagnosis, but the profound science of listening to, understanding and guiding the soul through its inner storms.* »

INTRODUCTION

Overview of psychiatry as a medical field.

Psychiatry, with all its mysteries and discoveries, is the fascinating branch of medicine that explores the depths of the human mind. From the dawn of our history, mankind has sought to understand the nature of disorders of the mind, those enigmas that seem at odds with visible physical injuries. Indeed, psychiatry, through its many metamorphoses, has devoted itself to the quest for these answers, navigating the meanders of consciousness, the unconscious, emotions and behaviour.

Psychiatry has always had a special place in the vast and varied field of medicine. Psychiatry is interested not only in the biology of the brain, but also in the impact of life experiences, cultures and societies on our mental health. It stands out for its ability to link body and mind, to recognise that our mental well-being is just as crucial as our physical health.

From ancient times, when mental illness was believed to be the result of the wrath of the gods, to the Renaissance, when asylums and hospices were the norm, psychiatry has evolved into the modern discipline that recognises, studies and treats mental disorders from both a scientific and a human perspective. It now uses advanced methods ranging from behavioural therapies to psychopharmacology, while remaining centred on the individual.

Psychiatry has also given rise to philosophical debates about the nature of reality, normality and otherness. What constitutes a healthy mental experience? How do we differentiate psychological suffering from normal variations in human experience? These questions lie at the heart of psychiatry and call for ongoing introspection, not just by healthcare professionals but by society as a whole.

As a medical field, psychiatry is a profoundly human, evolving and interdisciplinary adventure. It reminds us that caring for the mind is just as essential as caring for the body, and that it is our duty to continue to research, learn and evolve our understanding of this intangible but vital universe that is the human mind.

Importance of the nurse in a psychiatric ward.

At the heart of psychiatric care lies the nurse, an essential pillar in the dynamics of a multidisciplinary team. Their role is much more than simply carrying out medical tasks; psychiatric nurses are often the first line of interaction with patients, offering listening, understanding and support.

These care professionals operate in a world where communication and empathy are of paramount importance. Unlike other medical specialities, where symptoms can often be seen or measured, in psychiatry, suffering nestles in the intangible, in the intricacies of the mind and emotions. And that's where nurses come in with subtlety and finesse, using their training and intuition to assess and intervene, but also to build therapeutic relationships based on trust.

In addition, psychiatric nurses are trained to deal with potentially volatile or unpredictable situations. They are often confronted with crises that require a rapid, calm and informed response, whether to defuse an agitated patient or to provide immediate support to someone in deep distress.

In addition to managing emergencies, nurses play a fundamental role in patient care. They play an active role in drawing up care plans, coordinating with other healthcare professionals and implementing therapeutic interventions. Their role also extends to educating patients and their families, helping them to understand the disease, the treatment and how best to manage the situation on a day-to-day basis.

It should also be remembered that psychiatric nurses are often agents of change. By working directly in the field, they are able to observe shortcomings, needs and opportunities for improvement. In this way, they can contribute to innovation in psychiatric care, proposing new methods and approaches, always in the interests of the patient.

Ultimately, the psychiatric nurse embodies a delicate balance between science and humanity. They combine solid medical training with a deep understanding of their patients' emotional and psychological needs. Their importance in the field of psychiatry cannot be underestimated, as they play a key role in the healing, well-being and dignity of their patients.

Chapter 1:
HISTORY OF PSYCHIATRY
AND THE EVOLVING ROLE OF THE
NURSE

Treatment history mental illness.

The history of the treatment of mental illness is as old as the history of civilisation itself. It reflects the way in which different cultures and eras have understood and responded to mental suffering, ranging from superstition and stigmatisation to a more nuanced and compassionate understanding.

Antiquity:
In ancient times, mental illness was often attributed to supernatural causes, such as demonic possession or the wrath of the gods. Treatments ranged from exorcisms to religious rituals. However, figures such as Hippocrates in ancient Greece suggested that these illnesses could have physiological causes, advocating more natural approaches, such as dietary changes or rest.

The Middle Ages:
During the Middle Ages in Europe, the understanding of mental illness was largely influenced by religion. The Inquisition and the witch-hunt often targeted those perceived as mentally different. However, some places saw the emergence of asylums, although these were more places of isolation than true treatment centres.

Renaissance:
At the time of the Renaissance, there was a revival of interest in science and medicine. Despite this, conditions in

the asylums hardly changed, and many patients were mistreated or neglected.

18th and 19th centuries:
The Enlightenment brought a more humanitarian approach. Figures such as Philippe Pinel in France advocated more compassionate treatment of the mentally ill. In the United States, Dorothea Dix campaigned for the creation of asylums where patients could receive real care. It was also at this time that the concept of psychotherapy began to emerge.

20th century:
The discovery of antipsychotics in the 1950s marked a major turning point. These drugs enabled many patients to live a relatively normal life outside of institutions. Psychotherapy, particularly Freud's psychoanalysis, also gained in popularity.

However, the mid to late twentieth century saw a transition towards deinstitutionalisation, with care moving from hospitals to the community. This was both celebrated for promoting patient autonomy and criticised for leaving some without appropriate care.

21st century:
Today, the treatment of mental illness takes a holistic approach, combining medication, therapy, community interventions and recovery strategies. Stigma persists, but there is also growing recognition of the importance of mental health at all levels of society.

Over the centuries, the way in which society has perceived and treated mental illness has fluctuated between compassion and stigmatisation, between research and fear. This historical journey underlines the importance of continuing to seek more effective and humane ways of supporting those struggling with mental illness.

Evolution of the role
of the psychiatric nurse.

The changing role of the psychiatric nurse reflects the profound changes in the way society approaches and understands mental health. From simple caretaker to specialist therapist, the psychiatric nurse has undergone a remarkable transformation over the decades.

Origins:
In the early days of psychiatric asylums, nurses were often seen as guardians. Their main role was to maintain order, supervise patients and ensure the security of the institution. Training was minimal, and interventions were largely dictated by doctors.

Early 20th century:
With the rise of psychology and psychiatry as scientific disciplines, the psychiatric nurse began to play a more active role in the treatment of patients. Nurses were trained to observe and report on patient behaviour, administer medication and assist with therapies such as baths or electroconvulsive therapy.

Mid-twentieth century:
The introduction of antipsychotic drugs and the rise of psychotherapy brought new dimensions to the role of the nurse. Nurses were increasingly seen as essential members of the therapeutic team. Their training expanded, and they began to play an active role in developing and implementing treatment plans.

Late 20th century and early 21st century:
With the move towards deinstitutionalisation and community-centred care, psychiatric nurses found themselves at the forefront of community care. They took on case management, care coordination and the

supervision of drug treatment. Specialist nurses, or psychiatric nurse practitioners, acquired advanced skills in diagnosing, prescribing medication and providing therapy.

Nurses have also played a key role in mental health promotion, prevention and patient and community education. Their approach has also broadened to include not only the management of illness, but also support for recovery and the defence of patients' rights.

The evolving role of the psychiatric nurse is testament to the growing importance placed on mental health and the recognition of the central role nurses play in providing compassionate and specialist care. As psychiatry itself continues to evolve, it is clear that nurses will remain at the heart of this transformation, providing expertise, compassion and dedication every step of the way.

Impact of discoveries medical and scientific.

The history of psychiatry is closely linked to that of the medical and scientific discoveries that have shaped not only our understanding of mental illness, but also our methods of treatment. Each advance has had a profound impact on patients, practitioners and society as a whole.

1. Neurotransmitters:
The discovery of neurotransmitters, chemical substances that facilitate communication between neurons, revolutionised our understanding of brain function. This led to the formulation of theories on chemical imbalance as a potential cause of certain mental illnesses.

2. Psychotropic drugs:
The development of drugs such as antipsychotics, antidepressants and anxiolytics has radically transformed the treatment of mental illness. For example, the discovery of chlorpromazine in the 1950s enabled schizophrenia patients to live outside hospitals and ushered in the era of psychopharmacology.

3. Brain imaging techniques:
Tools such as MRI and PET scans have enabled researchers to observe the brain in action and identify the structural and functional differences associated with certain psychiatric disorders.

4. Cognitive behavioural therapies (CBT):
Based on sound scientific research, CBT has been shown to be effective in the treatment of many mental illnesses, helping patients to identify and change negative patterns of thought and behaviour.

5. Genetics and psychiatry:
Research into the heritability of certain mental illnesses has paved the way for molecular psychiatry. Although the exact origin of most mental disorders remains complex, it is now clear that there is a genetic component to conditions such as schizophrenia, bipolar disorder and depression.

6. Neuroplasticity:
The discovery that the brain can change and adapt throughout life, even in adulthood, has influenced approaches to rehabilitation and therapy, emphasising **the potential for recovery and growth.**

7. Biological treatments:
In addition to drugs, approaches such as electroconvulsive therapy (ECT), transcranial magnetic stimulation (TMS) and deep brain stimulation (DBS) have emerged as potentially

effective treatments for conditions resistant to other forms of intervention.

Each medical and scientific discovery has brought a new layer of understanding and opportunity to the field of psychiatry. These advances have not only improved outcomes for millions of patients, but have also helped to reduce the stigma associated with mental illness. Based on solid evidence, psychiatry continues to evolve, promising better interventions and a better quality of life for those suffering from mental disorders.

CHAPTER 2:
ANATOMY AND PHYSIOLOGY
OF THE BRAIN

Neurobiological basis
psychiatric disorders.

Neurobiology has proved to be a crucial field for deciphering the mysteries surrounding psychiatric disorders. While the exact mechanisms of many disorders are still poorly understood, some notable advances have enabled us to understand the neurobiological underpinnings of mental disorders.

1. Neurotransmitters:
It is widely accepted that neurotransmitter imbalances play a central role in many psychiatric disorders:
- **Depression**: Theories suggest that depression may result from an imbalance in certain neurotransmitters such as serotonin, noradrenaline and dopamine.
- **Schizophrenia: This is** associated with dopaminergic hyperactivity in certain areas of the brain.
- **Anxiety disorders**: These may be linked to an imbalance in the GABAergic system or in the neurotransmitter serotonin.

2. Cerebral circuits:
Disturbances in specific brain circuits are also suspected of being at the root of certain disorders:
- **Obsessive-compulsive disorder (OCD)**: Hyperactivity has been observed in the cingulo-striato-thalamo-cortical circuit.

- **Post-traumatic stress disorder (PTSD)**: Areas involved include the amygdala, medial prefrontal cortex and hippocampus.

3. Neuroplasticity:
Alterations in the brain's ability to form new connections and adapt may be linked to disorders such as depression. For example, reduced neuroplasticity in the hippocampus has been associated with depressive episodes.

4. Genetic aspects:
Genetics play a determining role in vulnerability to certain mental illnesses. Mutations or variations in specific genes can increase the risk of developing disorders such as schizophrenia, bipolar disorder or autism.

5. Inflammation and immunity:
Recent research suggests that an overactive immune response, leading to inflammation, may contribute to conditions such as depression and schizophrenia.

6. Environmental factors and neurobiology:
Traumatic experiences, particularly during crucial periods of development, can result in neurobiological changes. For example, childhood trauma can affect the size and function of the amygdala or hippocampus, contributing to disorders such as PTSD or attachment disorders.

The complexity of the human brain makes it extremely difficult to isolate the neurobiological causes of psychiatric disorders. Nevertheless, scientific advances have largely contributed to shedding light on certain fundamental mechanisms, enabling the development of more targeted and effective treatments. The ongoing integration of neurobiological, genetic and environmental discoveries is essential to improving the treatment and understanding of mental illnesses.

Interaction between the brain, neurotransmitters and psychotropic drugs.

The interaction between the brain, neurotransmitters and psychotropic drugs is at the heart of psychiatric pharmacology. To understand this complex exchange, it is essential to understand the basis of neuronal signalling and how drugs can influence these processes.

1. Neuronal communication and neurotransmitters:
The brain is made up of billions of neurons, and communication between them takes place mainly via synapses. At these junctions, chemical molecules called neurotransmitters are released by one neuron and received by another via specific receptors. This process triggers a series of electrical and chemical events that influence the functioning of the receptor neuron.

2. Neurotransmitter imbalance and mental illness:
Some psychiatric disorders are associated with neurotransmitter imbalances. For example, depression may be linked to a reduction in serotonin, noradrenaline or dopamine in certain parts of the brain.

3. Psychotropic drugs:
Psychotropic drugs intervene in this neuronal communication process, either by influencing the production, release, reception or degradation of neurotransmitters.
- **Antidepressants**: Most antidepressants, such as selective serotonin reuptake inhibitors (SSRIs), work by blocking the reuptake of serotonin, thereby increasing its availability at the synapse.
- **Antipsychotics**: These drugs, used mainly to treat schizophrenia, work by blocking dopamine receptors,

thereby reducing its action. Some new-generation antipsychotics also act on other neurotransmitters such as serotonin.

- **Anxiolytics**: Benzodiazepines, for example, increase the effect of GABA, an inhibitory neurotransmitter, producing a calming effect.
- **Mood stabilisers**: Drugs such as lithium, used to treat bipolar disorder, have a more complex mechanism of action which may involve several neurotransmitter systems.

4. Side effects and therapeutic implications:

As these drugs act on neurotransmitter systems, they can also cause side effects. For example, drugs that increase dopamine may improve mood or reduce psychotic symptoms, but may also cause involuntary movements or other undesirable effects. It is therefore crucial to adjust dosages and monitor patients in order to optimise therapeutic benefits while minimising side effects.

Understanding the interaction between the brain, neurotransmitters and psychotropic drugs is essential for modern psychiatry. It not only makes it possible to develop more effective treatments, but also to understand the biological basis of mental illness. As this knowledge develops, we can look forward to even more targeted interventions tailored to each individual, taking into account the nuances of the brain and its biochemistry.

Chapter 3:
DISORDERS
MAJOR PSYCHIATRIC DISORDERS

Classification of disorders (DSM-V).

The DSM-5, or "Diagnostic and Statistical Manual of Mental Disorders, Fifth Edition", is one of the major reference tools for mental health professionals in the United States and many other countries. It provides a classification of mental disorders and defines diagnostic criteria for each of them. Here is a simplified overview of the major categories of disorders defined in the DSM-5:

- Neurodevelopmental disorders: These are conditions that appear early in development. They include:
  - Autism spectrum disorder
  - Attention deficit hyperactivity disorder (ADHD)
  - Communication disorders
  - Specific learning   difficulties
- Psychotic disorders: These are characterised by changes in thinking, perceptions and/or behaviour.
  - Schizophrenia
  - Schizoaffective disorder
- Bipolar and related disorders:
  - Bipolar I and II disorder
  - Cyclothymia
- Depressive   disorders:
  - Major depressive   disorder
  - Dysthymic disorder (or persistent depressive disorder)
  - Substance/medication-induced depressive disorders

- Anxiety disorders:
  - Generalised anxiety   disorder
  - Panic disorder
  - Specific phobias
  - Social anxiety disorder
  - Separation anxiety   disorder
- Stress and trauma-related disorders:
  - Post-traumatic stress disorder (PTSD)
  - Acute stress disorder
  - Adjustment disorder
- Obsessive-compulsive disorder and related disorders:
  - Obsessive-compulsive disorder (OCD)
  - Hair-pulling disorder (trichotillomania)
  - Accumulation disorder
- Somatoform disorders:
  - Pain disorder
  - Somatic disorder linked to a functional form
- Eating disorders:
  - Anorexia nervosa
  - Nervous bulimia
  - Binge eating disorder
- Excretion disorders:
- Enuresis
- Encopresis
- Sleep and wakefulness disorders:
- Insomnia
- Narcolepsy
- Sleep apnoea syndrome
- Impaired sexual function:
- Erectile dysfunction
- Female sexual arousal disorder
- Gender identity dysmorphia.
- Substance use disorders and substance-induced disorders:
- Alcohol dependence
- Opioid use disorder
- Neurocognitive disorders:

27

- Major neurocognitive disorder (such as Alzheimer's disease)
- Mild neurocognitive disorder
- Personality disorders:
- Borderline personality disorder
- Antisocial personality disorder
- Avoidant personality disorder
- Other mental disorders.

It should be noted that this list is far from exhaustive and does not cover all the specific disorders or subtypes listed in the DSM-5. The manual strives to be a living tool, adapting in the light of new discoveries and clinical debates.

Symptoms, diagnosis and treatment of disorders such as schizophrenia, bipolarity, major depression, etc.

Let's look at the symptoms, diagnosis and treatment of these three major psychiatric disorders: schizophrenia, bipolar disorder and major depression.

1. Schizophrenia
Symptoms:
- **Positive symptoms**: hallucinations, delusions, disorganised thinking, agitated or bizarre behaviour.
- **Negative symptoms**: apathy, anhedonia (inability to feel pleasure), reduced emotional expression, difficulty initiating and sustaining activities.

Diagnosis:
Diagnosis is based on a clinical assessment including a history, mental examination and often brain imaging.
Treatment:

- **Antipsychotic medication**: can help manage positive symptoms.
- **Cognitive-behavioural therapy**: can help manage symptoms.
- **Rehabilitation programmes**: to help patients develop social and professional skills.

2. Bipolar disorder (Bipolarity)
Symptoms:
- **Manic phase**: exaggerated self-esteem, reduced need for sleep, excessive chatter, racing thoughts, distractibility, increase in focused activities (often with a grandiose perspective).
- **Depressive phase**: feelings of sadness or despair, loss of interest or pleasure in most activities, sleep disturbance, fatigue, feelings of worthlessness or excessive guilt, difficulty concentrating, thoughts of death or suicide.

Diagnosis:
- Based on a clinical assessment, including a detailed medical and psychiatric history.

Treatment:
- Mood stabilisers such as lithium.
- **Antipsychotics** to manage manic episodes.
- **Antidepressants** to treat depressive episodes.
- **Cognitive-behavioural therapy** to help identify and change negative behaviours and thoughts.

3. Major depression
Symptoms:
- Feelings of sadness or despair.
- Loss of interest or pleasure in activities.
- Changes in weight or appetite.
- Sleep disorders.
- Fatigue or loss of energy.
- Feelings of worthlessness.
- Difficulty concentrating.

- Suicidal thoughts or attempts.

Diagnosis:
- A thorough clinical assessment is necessary, with particular attention paid to the medical and psychiatric history.

Treatment:
- **Antidepressants**: There are several classes, such as SSRIs (selective serotonin reuptake inhibitors).
- **Cognitive-behavioural therapy** to help modify negative thoughts.
- **Electroconvulsive therapy (ECT):** used in severe cases where other treatments have failed.
- **Psychotherapy**: A variety of therapeutic modalities may be useful, depending on the patient's individual needs.

It is crucial to consult a mental health professional to obtain an accurate diagnosis and a suitable treatment plan. These summaries are general overviews and do not cover all aspects of each disorder.

Social impact and family problems.

Psychiatric disorders often have profound consequences not only for the individuals suffering from them, but also for their families, friends and society as a whole. Understanding these impacts can help raise awareness and strengthen support for patients and their families.

1. Social impact
- **Stigma and discrimination**: People with mental disorders can be stigmatised and discriminated against. This can limit their access to employment, housing or participation in social life.

- **Isolation**: Due to stigmatisation or symptoms such as social withdrawal or paranoia, these individuals may become isolated or shunned by society.
- **Occupational Problems**: Disorders can affect a person's ability to work or hold down a job, which can lead to financial instability.
- **Risky Behaviours**: Certain disorders, especially if left untreated, can increase the risk of dangerous or self-destructive behaviours, such as excessive alcohol or drug use, or criminal behaviour.
- **Access to care**: Stigma and lack of awareness can hamper access to appropriate and timely care.

2. Family impact
- **Relational tension**: Symptoms of a mental disorder, such as irritability or withdrawal, can cause tension or conflict within the family.
- **Emotional and Physical Burden**: Caring for a family member with a mental disorder can be emotionally and physically draining. This can lead to carer burnout.
- **Financial difficulties**: Mental health care can be expensive. If a family member is unable to work because of their illness, this can also have financial consequences for the household.
- **Education and awareness**: Family members often need to educate themselves about the disorder, which can take time and resources.
- **Impact on children**: If a parent suffers from a mental disorder, this can have an impact on their parenting role and, consequently, on the child's emotional and psychological well-being.
- **Changing family roles**: Roles and responsibilities within the family may change, for example, an adolescent may take on adult responsibilities to fill the void.

Recognising and understanding these impacts is essential to providing effective support to people with mental health problems and their families. With appropriate care, increased awareness and community support, many negative impacts can be mitigated or prevented.

Chapter 4:
PSYCHIATRIC ASSESSMENT TECHNIQUES

Clinical interviews.

The clinical interview in psychiatry is a fundamental part of patient assessment and management. It provides a framework in which the healthcare professional assesses, interacts and connects with the patient in order to establish a diagnosis, understand the patient's experience and plan appropriate treatment.

Main objectives of the clinical interview :
* Establishing a therapeutic relationship with the patient.
* Gather information on the symptoms present and their evolution, as well as the psychiatric, medical and social history.
* Assess the patient's current level of functioning.
* Assess the risks, particularly those associated with potential danger to yourself or others.
* Establish a diagnosis.
* Plan and discuss treatment options.

General structure of the clinical interview :
* **Introduction**: The clinician introduces him/herself, explains the purpose of the interview and establishes a secure and confidential environment.
* Case history :
    * **Identifiers** : Basic information such as name, age, occupation, etc.
    * **Reason for consultation**: Main reasons for the visit.

- **History of current illness**: detailed course of symptoms, duration, severity, triggering or mitigating factors.
- **Psychiatric history**: previous episodes, hospitalisations, treatments received, etc.
- **Medical and surgical history**: illnesses, medication, allergies, surgery.
- **Family history**: psychiatric or medical illnesses in the family, family dynamics.
- **Social history**: education, work, relationships, substance abuse, living environment.
- **Mental examination**: Structured assessment of the patient's current mental state. This includes appearance, attitude, mood, affect, thought flow, thought content (including delusions, hallucinations), perception, judgement, cognition, and suicidal/homicidal ideation.
- **Risk assessment**: Assessment of any imminent danger to self or others, need for hospitalisation or other emergency interventions.
- **Summary and diagnosis**: On the basis of the information gathered, the clinician formulates a provisional or definitive diagnosis.
- **Discussion of the Treatment Plan**: Clinician and patient discuss treatment options, expectations, benefits and associated risks.
- **Conclusion**: Summing up the main points, clarifying any questions or concerns the patient may have, and planning the next steps.

Clinical interviewing is both an art and a science. The ability to establish a relationship of trust, to ask the right questions, to listen actively and to interpret information is essential for an effective interview. In addition, it is important for clinicians to be aware of their own reactions and emotions during the interview and to be able to manage them appropriately.

Assessment scales and tests.

The use of assessment scales and tests in psychiatry is fundamental to quantifying, monitoring and comparing patients' symptoms. These standardised tools provide an objective means of assessing various facets of mental health, enabling clinicians to make more accurate assessments, monitor symptom progression over time and measure response to treatment. Here are some of the assessment scales and tests most commonly used in psychiatry:

1. Depression assessment scales :
   - **Hamilton Rating Scale for Depression (HAM-D)**: Used to assess the severity of depressive symptoms.
   - **Beck Depression Inventory (BDI):** Self-administered questionnaire assessing the presence and severity of depressive symptoms.
2. Anxiety assessment scales:
   - **Hamilton Anxiety Scale (HAM-A):** Used to assess the severity of anxiety symptoms.
   - **Beck Anxiety Scale (BAI):** Self-administered questionnaire measuring the severity of anxiety symptoms.
3. Schizophrenia assessment scales:
   - **Positive and Negative Assessment of Schizophrenia Scale (PANSS)**: Assesses the positive, negative and general symptoms of schizophrenia.
   - **Brief Psychopathology Rating Scale (BPRS):** Measures the severity of symptoms in various psychiatric illnesses, including schizophrenia.
4. Assessment of mania :
   - **Young Mania Rating Scale (YMRS)**: Used to measure the severity of manic symptoms.

5. Neuropsychological tests:
- **Mini-Mental State Examination (MMSE)**: Rapidly assesses overall cognitive functioning, often used to assess dementia.
- **Stroop test**: Assesses executive functions, particularly inhibition.
- **Rey-Osterrieth complex figure test**: Assesses visual memory and visuo-spatial functions.

6. Suicide risk assessment:
- **Beck hopelessness scale (BHS)**: Used to assess negative thoughts and feelings about the future.
- Beck Suicidal Ideation Scale (BIS): Assesses the severity of suicidal thoughts.

7. Assessment scales for attention disorders:
- **Adult Self-Report Scale for ADHD (ASRS-v1.1)**: Questionnaire designed to assess the symptoms of ADHD in adults.

8. Assessments of personality disorders:
- **Minnesota Multiphasic Personality Inventory (MMPI)**: Widely used to diagnose personality disorders and other psychiatric conditions.
- **Revised Millon Personality Inventory (MCMI-III)**: Assesses personality disorders and personality styles.

It is important to note that the use of these scales and tests must be carried out by trained professionals and as part of a full clinical assessment. These instruments provide valuable information which, when combined with a clinical assessment, can help inform diagnosis and treatment planning.

Behavioural observation.

Behavioural observation is a central pillar of psychiatry and clinical psychology. It provides a direct insight into how a patient behaves in different situations, offering essential information that may not be captured by other means, such as interviews or tests. Observation is particularly useful for patients who find it difficult to verbalise their emotions or who may not be aware of some of their behaviour.

1. Fundamental principles of behavioural observation:
   - **Objectivity:** The observer must strive to remain neutral and objective, avoiding interpreting or judging behaviour based on their own beliefs or feelings.
   - **Consistency:** Observation must be systematic and consistent. If several observers are involved, it is crucial that they are all trained in the same way.
   - **Context:** It is essential to take into account the context in which the behaviour takes place. For example, a patient may behave differently in a crowded waiting room than in a more intimate setting.
2. Key areas of observation in psychiatry:
   - **Physical appearance:** Dress, cleanliness, posture, facial expressions and any other notable aspect of the patient's appearance.
   - **Motor behaviour: Including** agitation, apathy, tics, tremors or other unusual movements.
   - **Social interaction:** how the patient interacts with others, whether they avoid eye contact, are distant or overly intrusive.
   - **Emotional reactivity:** How the patient reacts to stimuli, whether they appear emotionally flat or have exaggerated reactions.
   - **Verbalizations:** Not only what the patient says, but also how they say it: tone, volume, rate of speech.
   - **Specific symptoms:** Like hallucinations - a patient may appear to be listening or responding to voices that no-one else hears.
3. Applications of behavioural observation:
   - **Assessment:** Observation can help establish a diagnosis or determine the severity of a disorder.

- **Treatment planning:** Depending on the behaviours observed, specific interventions may be recommended.
- **Monitoring treatment:** Observing how a behaviour changes (or does not change) over time can help determine whether a treatment is effective.

4. Challenges and considerations:

- **Observer bias:** Observers may interpret behaviour through the prism of their own experiences and beliefs. Adequate training and regular checks can help to minimise this bias.
- **Reactivity:** Patients may change their behaviour because they know they are being observed. This is known as the observer effect.
- **Ethical considerations: It** is crucial that patients are informed and give their consent to be observed, and that their privacy is respected.

Behavioural observation is a valuable tool in the field of psychiatry. It provides a real-time overview of a patient's behaviour, complementing the information gathered by other means.

Chapter 5:
THE THERAPEUTIC RELATIONSHIP

Effective communication with the patient.

Communication with psychiatric patients is not just an exchange of information, but a delicate art that requires listening, empathy and respect. In this field, the way we communicate is often as important as what we say. Active listening is the cornerstone of this communication: it involves being fully present, focusing all your attention on the patient and rephrasing his or her words to make sure you have understood them correctly, while validating his or her feelings and concerns.

Open questioning is also essential. It encourages patients to talk freely about their experiences and emotions, creating a space where they feel heard and understood. This is all the more important in psychiatry, where patients may feel vulnerable or reluctant to share their most intimate thoughts.

But words are only part of the equation. Body language plays an equally crucial role. Appropriate eye contact, an open, relaxed posture and well-placed gestures can convey deep attention and genuine interest. Conversely, a closed posture or lack of eye contact can make the patient feel neglected or misunderstood.

Of course, clarification is sometimes necessary, especially in complex situations where it is crucial to avoid misunderstandings. However, it is essential to approach these moments with sensitivity, avoiding medical jargon and favouring clear, simple language.

Empathy and compassion, two fundamental qualities for any health professional, take on a particular dimension in psychiatry. Patients need to feel that they are not only being listened to, but understood and that their concerns are shared. That said, honesty and transparency are just as vital, especially when it comes to sensitive issues such as diagnosis, treatment and future prospects.

Finally, as well as being empathetic, you need to be careful to respect certain professional boundaries to ensure a healthy and constructive relationship. We must not forget that giving constructive feedback and managing our own emotions during these exchanges are also essential skills. After all, effective communication is a delicate balance between giving and receiving, understanding and being understood, all with the aim of providing the best possible care.

The importance of listening and empathy.

Listening and empathy are much more than simple communication skills, particularly in the medical field and, more specifically, in psychiatry. They are at the heart of the therapeutic relationship, anchoring the healthcare professional in a position not just of observer, but also of benevolent partner in the patient's therapeutic journey.

Listening, in its most authentic form, implies full and undivided attention. It requires putting aside one's own judgements, preconceived ideas and prepared responses to really hear what the patient is expressing. This listening goes beyond words. It picks up on tone, rhythm, silences and even what is not said. In a world where so many people feel misunderstood or ignored, being listened to can have immense therapeutic power.

Empathy, on the other hand, is the ability to put oneself in another person's shoes, to feel what they are feeling. It is not simple sympathy, which is compassion for the suffering of others. Empathy implies a deep understanding of the other person's emotions, thoughts and experiences. In psychiatry, this ability enables the professional to understand the patient's inner suffering, even when it is difficult to verbalise.

The importance of these two elements is manifold. **Firstly,** they create a safe space where patients can feel free to express their thoughts, emotions and concerns without fear of being judged. This feeling of safety can be fundamental to the healing process.

Secondly, listening and empathy foster trust. A patient who feels listened to and understood is more likely to cooperate with treatment, follow medical recommendations and express any concerns or uncertainties.

Thirdly, they provide a more complete picture of the patient. By listening carefully and showing empathy, the healthcare professional can identify key elements of the patient's history or experience that could influence the diagnosis or treatment plan.

Finally, listening and empathy humanise medicine. In a field where technology and protocols can sometimes eclipse the individual, these skills bring the focus back to the person behind the patient, reminding us that each individual is unique, with his or her own experiences, hopes and fears.

On the whole, listening and empathy are not simply tools among others, but rather the very essence of medical practice, strengthening the therapeutic relationship and facilitating the holistic healing of the individual.

Relationship challenges patient-nurse in psychiatry.

The patient-nurse relationship in psychiatry is an essential therapeutic alliance, but it is often fraught with challenges. Navigating the sometimes turbulent waters of mental health requires sensitivity, patience and resilience. Let's take a look at some of the main challenges inherent in this special relationship.

1. Stigmatisation of mental illness: Even in the medical environment, prejudices associated with psychiatry can persist. These attitudes may, consciously or unconsciously, influence the way nurses perceive and interact with patients, and vice versa.

2. Transference and counter-transference: These psychological phenomena can blur the therapeutic relationship. The patient may, for example, transfer to the nurse feelings he or she has towards another person in his or her life. Conversely, the nurse may feel irrational emotions towards the patient based on his or her own past experiences.

3. Complex communication: Certain mental disorders can impair a patient's ability to communicate clearly, whether due to mistrust, hallucinations, disorganised thinking or the severity of depression.

4. Unpredictable behaviour: Nurses may be confronted with situations where the patient becomes aggressive, self-destructive or unpredictable due to their mental state.

5. Resistance to treatment: Some patients may refuse medication or other interventions, either because they do not recognise their illness or because of unpleasant side effects.

6. Emotional exhaustion: Confronting psychological suffering on a daily basis can be emotionally draining for nurses. Compassion fatigue, a specific type of exhaustion, can set in.

7. Setting boundaries: Establishing and maintaining professional boundaries while being empathetic is crucial and can be a delicate balancing act.

8. Ethical decisions: Psychiatric nurses are sometimes faced with ethical dilemmas, such as respect for patient autonomy versus the need to intervene for the patient's safety or that of others.

9. Multidisciplinary collaboration: Working as part of a team with other professionals (psychiatrists, psychologists, social workers) can sometimes lead to disagreements over treatment or the direction of treatment.

10. Attachment and detachment: Forming a solid therapeutic bond without becoming too attached is essential. Too much distance can make the relationship cold, but excessive emotional investment can undermine the nurse's objectivity.

Whilst recognising these challenges, it is crucial to emphasise that the patient-nurse relationship in psychiatry also offers immense rewards. Moments of breakthrough, the development of trust and progress towards recovery can be deeply rewarding for the nurse and life-changing for the patient. Appropriate training, ongoing support and self-reflection are essential to successfully navigate this complex and rewarding relationship.

Chapter 6:
TECHNIQUES AND
TREATMENT METHODS

Individual and group therapy.

Both individual and group therapies are a fundamental pillar of psychiatric treatment. Each offers specific advantages and responds to different needs, although they can also complement each other. Let's take a closer look at these two forms of therapy, their characteristics, advantages and applications.

Individual therapies :
1. Features :
   * One-on-one interaction between patient and therapist.
   * A private environment that fosters a relationship of trust.
   * Customised to meet the patient's specific needs.
2. Advantages :
   * Intense focus on the patient's personal problems.
   * Allows you to deal with deeply private or sensitive subjects.
   * Flexibility in the therapeutic techniques used and the pace of sessions.
3. Common applications :
   * Cognitive behavioural therapy (CBT) to treat depression, anxiety, OCD, etc.
   * Psychodynamic therapy that explores unconscious conflicts and relational patterns.
   * Mindfulness-based therapies for stress and anxiety management.

Group therapies :
1. Features :
  * Several participants share their experiences under the guidance of one or more therapists.
  * The sessions take place in a structured environment.
  * The group offers an integrated support system.
2. Advantages :
  * Patients can feel less isolated by hearing the experiences of others.
  * Opportunity to learn social skills and receive feedback from peers.
  * The group offers a multiplicity of perspectives and potential solutions to a problem.
3. Common applications :
  * Support groups for specific problems such as addiction, bipolar disorder or eating disorders.
  * Talk therapy, where participants share their experiences and help each other.
  * Skills-based groups, such as social skills training or stress management groups.

The choice between individual or group therapy depends on the patient's specific needs, the nature of their problems and their personal preferences. In many cases, a combination of the two may be most beneficial, where individual therapy delves deeper into personal issues while group therapy offers community support and a variety of perspectives.

It is essential that the therapist or nurse assesses the patient correctly and guides them towards the treatment modality best suited to their condition and needs. Each modality, with its unique characteristics and benefits, has the potential to transform the patient's life and help them to move towards well-being and healing.

Drug treatment.

Drug treatment in psychiatry is a vast and complex field, playing a central role in the management of many mental disorders. Psychotropic drugs have revolutionised the treatment of psychiatric conditions, enabling many patients to lead more normal and functional lives. Here is a fluid overview of drug treatment in psychiatry.

In the corridors of hospitals and psychiatrists' surgeries, drug treatment is often evoked as a beacon of hope for those struggling with mental turmoil. Since the discovery of the first antipsychotics in the 1950s, the landscape of psychiatry has been profoundly transformed. The drugs have become invaluable allies, restoring hope and independence to millions of people around the world.

1. Classes of medicines :
- **Antidepressants:** Used to treat depression, they work by balancing neurotransmitters in the brain. SSRIs (selective serotonin reuptake inhibitors) such as Prozac are commonly used.
- **Antipsychotics:** These drugs are prescribed to treat the symptoms of schizophrenia and other psychotic disorders. They may be first-generation, such as haloperidol, or new-generation, such as olanzapine.
- **Mood stabilisers:** Prescribed mainly for bipolar disorder, they regulate mood swings. Lithium is a well-known mood stabiliser.
- **Anxiolytics:** Benzodiazepines are used to treat anxiety and panic disorders. However, they should be used with caution because of their habit-forming potential.
- **Stimulants:** These are mainly prescribed to treat ADHD (attention deficit hyperactivity disorder). Ritalin is one example.

2. The therapeutic decision: The decision to prescribe a drug must be meticulous. It is based on a thorough clinical assessment, an understanding of the patient's medical history, and the potential benefits of the treatment in relation to the risks.

3. Side-effects: All medicines have side-effects, some minor, others more serious. Regular monitoring is essential to ensure that the patient tolerates the treatment well and that the benefits outweigh the risks.

4. Therapeutic adherence: One of the major challenges is to ensure that patients take their medication regularly. Forgetfulness, concerns about side effects or a lack of understanding of the treatment can lead to non-adherence.

5. The role of the healthcare team : Nurses play an essential role in educating patients about their medicines, monitoring side effects, and encouraging adherence. Their role is just as crucial as that of the prescriber.

6. Combined treatment: In many cases, a combined approach combining medication and psychotherapy is the most effective. The therapeutic alliance, reinforced by medication and emotional support, can offer the best results.

Advances in drug treatment in psychiatry continue to grow, offering new possibilities and hope. However, it is vital to understand that medication is only one tool in the vast therapeutic toolbox available to treat mental disorders. A holistic approach, taking into account the patient's physical, emotional, social and mental well-being, is the key to successful treatment.

Alternative therapies and complementary (art therapy, music therapy).

Alternative and complementary therapies are playing an increasingly important role in the field of mental health. Far from replacing conventional treatments, these approaches are intended to complement them, offering an additional dimension to patient care. Let's look at how these therapies, through the prism of creativity and expression, can play a life-saving role in the healing process.

In the vast world of psychiatry, each individual is a world unto himself, with his own means of expression, obstacles and resources. While drugs and traditional therapies are the mainstays of treatment, other, less conventional but equally powerful approaches have found their way into the field: alternative and complementary therapies.

Art therapy :
Art, in all its many facets, is a window onto the soul.
1. The creative process: In art therapy, the act of creating is central. Painting, drawing, sculpting: every movement, every choice of colour or shape becomes an extension of the emotion, of the feeling.
2. Benefits: It provides a space for free expression, where words may fail. Traumas, fears and hopes are translated into works of art, raising awareness and externalising problems.
3. Applications: Art therapy has been shown to be effective in a wide range of situations, including autism spectrum disorders, trauma, depression and dementia.

Music therapy :
Music, that universal art, resonates within us all, awakening emotions and memories.

1. Listening and creating: In music therapy, listening to music can provoke emotional reactions, as can creating melodies or rhythms.

2. Benefits: It promotes relaxation, reduces anxiety, improves self-esteem and enhances social skills. It can also stimulate memory in people with neurodegenerative disorders.

3. Applications : Music therapy is used for a variety of conditions, from schizophrenia and depression to neurological disorders and paediatric conditions.

Alternative and complementary therapies do not seek to replace traditional interventions, but rather to enrich the therapeutic pathway. In these safe spaces, patients are invited to reconnect with themselves, to explore new ways of expressing their pain, hopes and desires. Art and music, in their universal languages, offer bridges to healing, reminding us that well-being is a symphony of many instruments.

Chapter 7:
CRISIS MANAGEMENT

Recognition warning signs.

Recognising warning signs in psychiatry is essential. These warning signs, often subtle manifestations of underlying changes, can be the prelude to a crisis or an exacerbation of an existing mental disorder. Early detection not only enables rapid intervention, but also better management of the situation, and even prevention of more severe crises.

Imagine yourself walking through a magnificent garden. Everything seems serene and peaceful, then suddenly a shadow looms, heralding a possible storm. In the same way, in the complex garden of the human mind, certain discreet signs can presage internal storms.

1. Mood swings :
Even before clinical symptoms become apparent, unusual mood fluctuations may be noticed. A normally calm patient may become irritable or, conversely, a normally cheerful person may sink into a persistent gloom.
2. Behavioural changes :
Changes in daily habits, such as sleep, appetite or personal hygiene, are often warning signs. Social isolation, reduced interaction or avoidance of situations previously enjoyed can also be revealing.
3. Altered speech :
Difficulty following a conversation, disorganised thinking or rapid, disjointed speech may indicate an underlying problem.

4. Somatic symptoms :
Inexplicable physical complaints, such as frequent headaches, abdominal pain or persistent fatigue, can sometimes reflect a psychiatric disorder.

5. Increased sensitivity :
Excessive reactivity to stimuli, whether auditory, visual or emotional, can also be a warning sign.

6. Perceptual disorders :
Auditory or visual hallucinations, however slight, or a feeling of disconnection from reality, as in dissociative states, should be taken seriously.

7. Negative thoughts :
Persistent dark thoughts, obsessions, thoughts of death or irrational preoccupations can herald a crisis.

Recognising warning signs does not necessarily mean that a crisis is imminent, but it does underline the importance of increased vigilance. For healthcare professionals and their loved ones alike, it is essential to listen, observe and communicate. By anticipating and recognising these signs, we can create a safe environment for the patient, facilitate access to appropriate care and, often, prevent the progression to more critical situations. In the delicate ballet of mental health, prevention is a dance in which every step counts.

Intervention techniques in the event of aggression or a suicide attempt or self-aggression.

When faced with emergency situations in psychiatry, such as aggression, attempted suicide or self-aggression, the response of professionals must be rapid, appropriate and based on proven principles of intervention. These situations require specific skills, appropriate training and sharp clinical judgement to ensure the safety of the patient and the care team.

Navigating the stormy waters of psychiatric crises requires self-control, a controlled sense of urgency and honed interpersonal skills.

1. Assessment of the situation :
Before any intervention, it is essential to quickly assess the seriousness of the situation and the level of danger for the patient, staff and other patients.

2. Verbal communication :
Using a calm, reassuring voice, clear language and active listening can defuse many tense situations. Making eye contact, speaking from a safe distance and using reformulation techniques can help create a connection with the patient.

3. Safety zone :
It is vital to ensure that the immediate environment is safe. This may mean removing potentially dangerous objects or placing the patient in a safe room.

4. De-escalation techniques :
These techniques include empathic listening, assertion, clarification, offering choices where possible, and setting clear and consistent boundaries.

5. Physical intervention :
If the patient represents an immediate threat to themselves or others, and verbal techniques have not worked, physical intervention may be necessary. This should always be carried out by trained staff, using non-violent techniques and as little force as possible.

6. Drug administration :
In certain situations, medication may be administered to calm the patient. This should always be done in accordance with established medical protocols and under clinical supervision.

7. Post-intervention evaluation :
Once the crisis has been resolved, a full assessment of the patient is crucial to determine the triggering factors, assess future risks and adjust the treatment plan.
8. Team support :
Crisis situations can be traumatic for staff. It is therefore essential to provide a space for debriefing, supervision and support for the team members involved.

Dealing with a crisis in psychiatry requires a fusion of clinical skills, human empathy and professional judgement. It is a delicate balance between responding to the urgency of the moment and preserving the patient's dignity and rights. In these tense moments, the ultimate goal is always the patient's safety and well-being, and the prevention of future crises.

The importance of de-escalation and restraint.

De-escalation and restraint are two crucial methods for managing emergency situations in psychiatry, particularly when a patient presents a risk to themselves or others. Understanding their importance helps us to better understand the global and ethical approach to treating patients in crisis situations.

The world of psychiatry can sometimes seem like a turbulent ocean, with waves of emotion, currents of thought and storms of behaviour. In this environment, de-escalation and restraint play a vital role in restoring calm and ensuring safety.

1. De-escalation: The power of words
  - **Reducing the danger:** When a patient becomes agitated, verbal de-escalation aims to prevent an

escalation of aggression, avoiding the need for physical intervention.
- **Preserving dignity:** De-escalation means treating patients with respect and dignity, acknowledging their emotional experience while seeking to reassure them.
- **Human connection:** Through communication, we try to establish an empathic connection with the patient, by understanding their needs and reassuring them about the treatment.

2. Restraint: An extreme measure
- **Last resort:** Physical or chemical restraint is a heavy intervention that should only be used as a last resort, when all other methods have failed and the patient represents an imminent danger.
- **Limited duration:** Restraint must be as short as possible, always aiming to return to a state where the patient can be managed without physical or chemical restrictions.
- **Protection:** Its primary objective is to protect patients from themselves, healthcare staff and other patients.

3. The interconnection of the two methods :
It is essential to understand that these two methods are not mutually exclusive. De-escalation can be used in combination with more restrictive methods. For example, even when a patient is in restraint, verbal de-escalation efforts should continue in order to reduce their anxiety and reassure them.

De-escalation and restraint are not simply technical tools, but part of an ethical and humane approach. They are a reminder of the importance of approaching patients in crisis with compassion, respect and professionalism. The ultimate goal is always to guarantee safety while preserving the patient's dignity. In the tumultuous journey of psychiatric recovery, these methods serve as beacons, guiding both patient and carer towards calmer waters.

CHAPTER 8:
ETHICS AND PROFESSIONAL CONDUCT IN PSYCHIATRY

Patients' rights.

Patients' rights in psychiatry are a central pillar of contemporary medical practice. Despite the sometimes complex nature of psychiatric care, it is crucial that every patient is treated with dignity, respect and within the framework of a clearly defined ethical process.

At the heart of the complex labyrinth of psychiatry, the light of respect and dignity guides every decision taken. Patients' rights are that light, ensuring that every individual, despite the challenges they may face, is treated with the humanity and respect they deserve.

1. Right to information :
Every patient has the right to understand the nature of their illness, the proposed treatments and the possible alternatives. This information must be provided in a clear, accessible manner and in a language that the patient can understand.

2. Right to informed consent :
Before any medical intervention, patients must give their consent after being informed of the risks, benefits and alternatives of the treatment.

3. Right to confidentiality :
Patients' medical information is confidential. It can only be shared with the patient's consent or if required by law to protect the individual or others.

4. Right to respect for dignity and non-discrimination :
Regardless of race, religion, gender, sexual orientation or socio-economic status, every patient must be treated with equality and respect.

5. Right to appropriate treatment :
Every patient has the right to receive high-quality care, based on current medical knowledge and tailored to their individual needs.

6. Right to liberty and security :
Restrictions on freedom, such as restraint or forced hospitalisation, should only be used as a last resort and for the shortest possible time.

7. Right to refuse treatment :
Unless there is an immediate risk to the life of the patient or others, every patient has the right to refuse treatment, even if it is recommended by a healthcare professional.

8. Right to lodge a complaint :
If a patient feels that their rights have been violated or that they have not received appropriate care, they have the right to lodge a complaint with the relevant authorities.

9. Right to regular review of treatment :
Especially in the case of long-term treatment or hospitalisation, it is crucial to regularly review the appropriateness and effectiveness of the treatment.

In the world of psychiatry, where the boundaries between mental health and illness can often seem blurred, patients' rights serve as an unfailing guide. They remind healthcare professionals of their duty to each individual, ensuring that medical practice is ethical, respectful and patient-centred. The journey to recovery is a partnership between patient and carer, where trust, respect and dignity are the cornerstones.

Confidentiality and professional secrecy.

Confidentiality and professional secrecy are a fundamental pillar of the therapeutic relationship in medicine, and in psychiatry in particular. These principles guarantee emotional security, enabling patients to confide freely in the knowledge that their information will not be divulged.

In the sanctuary of medical consultations, patients reveal their fears, hopes, pains and dreams. The silent promise that hangs in the air is that of professional secrecy: a guarantee that what is said within these walls remains within these walls.

1. The importance of confidentiality :
Confidentiality is the foundation on which patient-provider trust is built. It allows patients to share their concerns openly without fear of judgement or disclosure. In a psychiatric context, where introspection and vulnerability are often necessary for treatment, confidentiality is crucial.

2. The boundaries of professional secrecy :
Professional secrecy extends far beyond simply not sharing information. It is an ethical and legal duty that prevents healthcare professionals from divulging information about a patient without their explicit consent.

3. Exceptions to the rule :
Although confidentiality is paramount, it is not absolute. There are exceptions, notably when the patient represents an imminent danger to himself or to others, or when the law explicitly requires the disclosure of information (as in the case of certain infectious diseases).

4. Technological issues and confidentiality :
With the advent of digital technology and the growing use of electronic medical records, the issue of security and confidentiality of patient data is becoming increasingly important. Protecting data against hacking or leaks has become a major challenge.

5. The patient's role in confidentiality :
It is important that patients understand their rights in terms of confidentiality. This includes the right to know who has access to their information, how it is used and stored, and how it can be shared.

Confidentiality and professional secrecy are more than just rules or guidelines; they reflect the deep respect and duty of care that healthcare professionals have for their patients. In the complex theatre of psychiatry, where emotions, memories and traumas are often laid bare, this promise of discretion helps to establish a solid therapeutic relationship based on mutual trust and respect.

Ethical dilemmas specific to psychiatry.

Ethical dilemmas in psychiatry are deeply rooted in the tension between the health professional's duty of care and respect for patient autonomy. In this particular field of medicine, where the mind and identity are directly concerned, these issues take on added importance.

The world of psychiatry is a place of paradoxes. It is a place where intangible pain manifests itself visibly, where the struggle for mental clarity can often blur ethical lines. Let's look at some of these ethical dilemmas specific to psychiatry:

1. Involuntary hospitalisation :
When, and to what extent, is it ethical to forcibly confine a patient? If a patient is perceived to be a danger to himself or others, hospitalisation may be justified. However, determining what constitutes a "danger" is subjective and can be controversial.

2. Forced treatment :

Administering medicines or therapies to patients against their will is a subject of intense debate. While this may be in the patient's best interests, it raises the question of individual autonomy versus **overall** well-being.

3. Decision-making capacity :

How can we assess whether a patient is capable of making informed decisions about their treatment? And if not, who should make these decisions for them?

4. Confidentiality versus protection :

If a patient confides that they intend to harm themselves or others, the healthcare professional is faced with a dilemma: respect confidentiality or intervene to protect the patient or a third party.

5. Dualist relationships :

The therapist and patient may have multiple relationships (for example, the therapist could also be a friend or colleague). How can these relationships be managed without compromising the integrity of the treatment?

6. Use of restraints :

The use of physical methods to control agitated patients is controversial. Although sometimes necessary for safety, they can be perceived as inhumane or traumatic.

7. Treatment of gender identity spectrum disorders :

The treatment of individuals suffering from gender dysphoria, particularly minors, is a subject of ethical debate. How do we balance respect for the patient's identity with medical and psychological concerns?

Navigating the sometimes troubled waters of psychiatry requires a solid ethical compass. Ethical dilemmas remind healthcare professionals that they must constantly balance the imperatives of the duty of care with respect for patient dignity and autonomy. In this delicate dance, the key lies in communication, reflection and commitment to the well-being of each individual.

Chapter 9:
THE WORK
IN A MULTIDISCIPLINARY TEAM

Role and functions
of different professionals.

The psychiatric service does not rely solely on the work of psychiatrists. It is a collaborative orchestration involving a multitude of professionals. Each, with his or her own speciality and expertise, contributes to the overall, holistic care of the patient.

1. The psychiatrist :
Psychiatrists specialise in the diagnosis, treatment and prevention of mental disorders. Their training enables them to prescribe medication, recommend therapies and intervene in situations requiring hospitalisation.
- Main functions:
- Diagnostic assessment.
- Prescription of psychotropic drugs.
- Supervision of treatment plans.

2. The Psychiatric Nurse :
Nurses are often the first point of contact for patients. They play a crucial role in the day-to-day management of care, administering medication and observing patients.
- Main functions:
- Direct patient care.
- Administration of medicines.
- Monitoring behaviour and symptoms.
- Educating patients about their treatment.

3. The Clinical Psychologist :
The psychologist focuses on psychotherapy and psychological assessment, offering insights into the patient's behaviour, emotions and thoughts.
- Main functions:
- Individual, family or group psychotherapy.
- Psychological assessments.
- Setting up intervention programmes.

4. The Social Worker :
This professional helps patients to manage and understand their illnesses, while connecting them with external resources and supporting their social needs.
- Main functions:
- Psychosocial support.
- Liaison with community resources.
- Advice on employee rights and benefits.

5. The Occupational Therapist :
Occupational therapists focus on improving patients' day-to-day skills, enabling them to lead as independent a life as possible.
- Main functions:
- Assessment of functional capabilities.
- Setting up therapeutic activities.
- Training in daily living skills.

6. The Clinical Pharmacist :
Specialising in psychotropic drugs, the pharmacist advises the team on side effects, drug interactions and appropriate therapeutic regimens.
- Main functions:
- Monitoring medication.
- Advice on therapeutic diets.
- Educating patients about medicines.

7. The Psychomotrician :

This professional focuses on the relationship between the psychological and motor aspects of the patient, using movement as a means of expression and therapy.

- Main functions:
- Movement therapy.
- Assessment of body tensions and blockages.
- Relaxation and body techniques.

The richness of the psychiatry department lies in the diversity of its staff. This multidisciplinary approach makes it possible to address the many facets of mental disorders, offering patients comprehensive, individualised care. In this therapeutic ecosystem, each professional makes his or her own contribution, working in symbiosis for the well-being of the patient.

Collaboration and effective communication within the team.

Collaboration and communication within the psychiatry team are essential to guarantee high-quality patient care. This inter-professional collaboration enables the different areas of expertise to be combined to provide holistic care. It's a delicate ballet, in which each member plays a crucial role, requiring fluid communication to function smoothly.

The field of psychiatry is rich in complexity. Each patient is an enigma, with unique symptoms, histories, hopes and fears. Faced with this complexity, teamwork becomes a key element. But how does this collaboration come to life?

1. Coordination meetings :

These are regular meetings where team members share patient updates, discuss progress, concerns and treatment strategies. These meetings allow the team to stay on the same wavelength and work in a consistent manner.

2. Documentation Claire :
Keeping clear, detailed and up-to-date records is essential. This enables each member of the team to have access to the information they need to understand the patient's progress and to adjust their interventions accordingly.

3. Respect for Roles :
Each professional brings specific expertise. Respecting and valuing each person's role builds trust within the team and encourages closer collaboration.

4. Communication tools :
The use of modern technological tools, such as electronic medical record management systems and secure communication applications, can greatly facilitate the exchange and sharing of information between members.

5. Joint training :
Interprofessional training can help to strengthen communication skills, understand each other's roles and responsibilities, and build a culture of collaboration.

6. Constructive feedback :
Effective communication also requires the ability to give and receive feedback. This is a learning opportunity, where members can share suggestions, concerns and praise in a constructive way.

7. Conflict Resolution :
Disagreements are inevitable. However, proactive and positive conflict management, with the emphasis on listening and finding common solutions, ensures that differences do not adversely affect the quality of care.

Communication and collaboration in psychiatry are not just a question of logistics. They reflect a philosophy of care that recognises that mental health is complex and multifactorial. By working together, sharing knowledge and valuing each other's contributions, the team can offer care that is greater than the sum of its parts. In this collaborative dance, every step, every movement, every gesture counts, making harmony a tangible reality.

CHAPTER 10:
PREVENTION AND EDUCATION

The role of the nurse
in relapse prevention.

Relapse is a major concern in the treatment of mental disorders. A relapse can be defined as the return of symptoms of a disorder after a period of remission or improvement. For patients, their families and healthcare professionals, relapse can be a destabilising and painful experience, marked by deterioration in functionality, disruption of daily life and often hospitalisation.

In this context, the psychiatric nurse plays a fundamental role in relapse prevention. As the central pillar of the continuum of care, nurses are well placed to identify warning signs, educate patients and intervene proactively.

1. Patient education :
The nurse educates patients about their illness, the risk factors for relapse, and the importance of adhering to treatment. A better understanding of the disease enables the patient to recognise the warning signs and take preventive measures.

2. Medication monitoring :
Ensuring that patients take their medication correctly is crucial. Nurses can advise on the management of side effects, regularity of intake and coordination with the pharmacist to ensure that medicines are available.

3. Clinical observation :
The nurse closely observes the patient's behaviour, mood and symptoms. Any subtle changes could be an indicator of a potential relapse.

4. Promoting Healthy Lifestyles :
A balanced lifestyle is a key element in prevention. Nurses encourage healthy habits such as a balanced diet, regular physical activity, good sleep and limiting the use of psychoactive substances.

5. Stress management :
Stress is a common trigger. Nurses can introduce stress management techniques such as meditation, relaxation or cognitive behavioural therapy.

6. Liaison with Family and Friends :
The family can be a valuable ally in preventing relapses. The nurse makes the family aware of the warning signs and involves them in the care plan.

7. Psychosocial support :
In addition to medical interventions, social support is essential. Nurses can refer patients to support groups or community resources.

8. Crisis plans :
Together with the patient, the nurse draws up an action plan in the event of significant deterioration, detailing the steps to be taken, the people to contact and the emergency measures.

The role of the nurse in relapse prevention is dynamic, multifaceted and crucial. Through their targeted interventions, their closeness to the patient and their holistic vision of care, nurses are a bulwark against relapse, ensuring that every patient can live their life with resilience, hope and autonomy.

Patient education and their families.

Educating patients and their families about mental health is fundamental to successful recovery. It is a process that goes beyond the simple transmission of information; it aims to empower patients and those around them, reinforce their understanding and give them the tools they need to manage their illness on a day-to-day basis. Because of their central position in the care team, nurses are often the main educators.

Understanding as a Starting Point :
Any educational approach in psychiatry begins with an empathetic understanding of the patient's reality. By recognising the feelings, concerns and aspirations of the patient and his or her family, the nurse can develop an appropriate educational strategy.

1. Information on the disease :
   - **Nature and symptoms:** Explain the disease, its typical symptoms and how it may develop.
   - **Causes:** Identify the biological, genetic, environmental and psychosocial factors likely to contribute to the disease.
   - **Treatments available:** Medication, therapies, psychosocial interventions.

2. Importance of Treatment Adherence :
   - **Clarification on medicines:** How they work, why they are prescribed, possible side effects.
   - **Adherence:** Discuss barriers to taking medication regularly and techniques for improving adherence.

3. Recognition of Warning Signs :
Educate people about the warning signs of a relapse or exacerbation of symptoms, and the importance of early intervention.

4. Stress Management Skills :
Introduce relaxation techniques, meditation or other strategies to manage stress, a major risk factor for many psychiatric disorders.

5. Mental Health Promotion :
- **Lifestyle habits:** The importance of a healthy diet, physical exercise and regular sleep.
- **Avoiding substances:** The dangers of alcohol, drugs and other substances in relation to illness.

6. Role and Support of the Family :
- **Active listening:** Teaching family members to listen without judging.
- **Intervention:** How to intervene appropriately when the patient is in crisis.

7. Resources and Support Networks :
Referrals to support groups, associations and other community resources.

Educating patients and their families is a journey. It requires patience, repetition and adjustment to the changing needs of the patient. As educators, nurses strive not only to impart knowledge, but also to instil hope, build resilience and encourage autonomy. In the complex maze of psychiatry, this education becomes the compass that guides the patient and his or her family towards a balanced and fulfilled life.

The importance of raising awareness the general public.

In a world where mental illness continues to be shrouded in stigma and misunderstanding, raising public awareness is of paramount importance. It's not just about disseminating information, but also about changing perceptions, attitudes and behaviours towards those living with mental disorders. Let's look at why this is essential and how it impacts society as a whole.

Dispelling Myths and Stigmas:
Mental illness is often shrouded in myth and prejudice, fuelled by ignorance, fear and sometimes biased media portrayals. These stigmas can lead to discrimination, isolation and shame for sufferers. Raising awareness among the general public means offering a more accurate and nuanced picture of mental disorders, which can help to reduce these stigmas.

Mental Health Promotion :
Raising awareness does not just mean talking about illnesses, but also promoting good mental health. This includes lifestyle habits that promote psychological well-being, the importance of listening to others and mutual support in communities.

Making it easier to find help :
Many people hesitate to seek help for fear of judgement. Raising public awareness creates an environment where individuals feel more comfortable talking about their mental challenges and seeking help without hesitation.

Influencing Public Policy :
An informed and aware public is more likely to support policies favourable to mental health, whether in terms of funding, research or prevention programmes. This positive pressure from the public can lead political decision-makers to prioritise mental health in their agendas.

Creating a More Empathetic Society :
Awareness-raising helps to cultivate a society where empathy and understanding are valued. In such a society, people with mental health problems are seen not as "others", but as integral members of the community, entitled to respect, support and dignity.

Preventive Education :
By raising public awareness of the early signs of mental disorders, we can encourage early intervention, thereby reducing the severity and duration of the illness. It's an investment in the future, because prevention is often more cost-effective than treatment.

Raising public awareness of mental health is a crucial task that goes beyond simply providing information. It is a societal movement aimed at building a world where mental illness is understood, not stigmatised, and where support is available to all. For mental health professionals, including nurses, raising awareness is not only a professional duty, but also an act of humanity, aimed at building bridges of understanding in a diverse and interconnected society.

Chapter 11:
PSYCHOPHARMACOLOGY
IN DETAIL

Mechanisms of
psychotropic drugs action

Psychotropic drugs play a central role in the treatment of many mental illnesses. These drugs act by modifying the activity of neurotransmitters in the brain. To understand the mechanism of action of psychotropic drugs, it is essential to look first at neurotransmitters, the molecules that act as chemical messengers in the nervous system.

The Role of Neurotransmitters :
The brain is a complex network of interconnected neurons. To communicate with each other, these neurons use molecules called neurotransmitters. These are released by one neuron, cross a small gap called a synapse, and bind to specific receptors on another neuron. This process influences a multitude of functions, from mood regulation to motor coordination.

How Psychotropic Drugs Work :
Psychotropic drugs act by altering the quantity or activity of certain neurotransmitters. Here are a few examples of their mechanisms of action:
- **Selective serotonin reuptake inhibitors (SSRIs):** Used mainly to treat depression, SSRIs increase the concentration of serotonin in the synapse by reducing its reuptake by neurons.
- **Antipsychotics:** These drugs, used to treat disorders such as schizophrenia, often work by

blocking the receptors for dopamine, a key neurotransmitter in the reward and motivation circuits.

- **Mood stabilisers**: For example, lithium, used in bipolar disorder, influences several neurotransmitters and cell signalling pathways. Its exact mechanism of action is still under investigation.
- **Benzodiazepines**: Prescribed for anxiety and sleep disorders, they increase the effectiveness of GABA, an inhibitory neurotransmitter that reduces neuronal activity.
- **Stimulants**: Used to treat attention deficit hyperactivity disorder (ADHD), they increase levels of dopamine and noradrenaline in the brain.

The Complexity of Psychotropic Drug Action :
It is important to note that the action of psychotropic drugs is complex. The same drug may have several mechanisms of action, and patients may react differently to the same treatment. What's more, the balance between therapeutic benefits and side effects varies from one individual to another.

Understanding the mechanisms of action of psychotropic drugs is essential for optimal patient care. This enables healthcare professionals, particularly nurses, to administer treatments in an informed manner, to educate patients about their medication, and to observe and report any side effects or drug interactions. In a field where each molecule can have a profound impact on a patient's quality of life, this understanding is at the heart of clinical practice.

Managing side effects.

Managing the side effects of psychotropic drugs is a crucial aspect of psychiatric treatment. Although these drugs are effective for many patients, they can also cause a range of undesirable effects, from mild to severe. Ensuring proper monitoring, educating patients and adapting treatments can greatly improve patient well-being and compliance.

Understanding side effects:
Each psychotropic drug has its own side-effect profile. For example, some antipsychotics can cause weight gain or involuntary movements, while some antidepressants can cause gastrointestinal or sexual problems.

Patient Education :
The first step in managing these effects is to educate the patient. Patients need to be informed about possible side effects, their frequency and severity, and the signs to look out for. This helps them to identify a potential problem quickly and to consult their carer.

Regular Surveillance :
Regular monitoring, through consultations and analyses, is essential to detect and manage side effects. For example, blood tests may be necessary to monitor the effects of mood stabilisers on the kidneys or thyroid.

Management strategies :
- **Adjusting doses:** Reducing the dose can often alleviate side effects without compromising the effectiveness of the drug.
- **Changing medication:** If a patient does not tolerate a medication, another medication in the same or a different class can be tried.
- **Adjunctive medication:** In some cases, another drug may be added to counter a specific side effect.
- **Scheduling:** Sometimes, simply by changing the time you take your medication, you can minimise side effects.

- **Non-drug support:** For certain side effects, such as weight gain, dietary support or physical therapy may be beneficial.

Effective Communication :
Encouraging patients to communicate openly about their symptoms and concerns is vital. Sometimes a side effect can be embarrassing or uncomfortable for the patient, and they may not mention it unless asked directly.

Managing side effects is a delicate task that requires close collaboration between the patient and the healthcare professional. Nurses, as first responders and day-to-day carers, play a central role in this management. They must not only actively monitor these effects, but also offer support, education and guidance, ensuring that psychiatric treatment is not only effective, but also safe and well tolerated.

Drug interactions.

Drug interactions are changes in the effect of a drug due to the presence of another drug, food or substance. They can potentiate or inhibit the action of a drug, leading to reduced efficacy or an increased risk of side effects. In the field of psychiatry, where many patients may be taking several drugs at the same time, understanding and managing drug interactions is essential.

Types of Drug Interactions :
- **Pharmacodynamic interactions:** These occur when two drugs act at the same site in the body and have similar or opposite effects. For example, a sedative antidepressant and an anxiolytic may have an additive effect, leading to excessive sedation.

- **Pharmacokinetic interactions:** These occur when one drug affects the absorption, distribution, metabolism or excretion of the other drug. For example, one drug may inhibit an enzyme that metabolises another drug, thereby increasing its concentration in the body.

Consequences of Interactions :

- **Reduced Therapeutic Effects:** A drug interaction may reduce the efficacy of a drug, thereby compromising treatment.
- **Increased side effects:** Interactions can also increase the undesirable or toxic effects of a drug.

Prevention and Management :

- **Complete assessment:** When prescribing, the healthcare professional must have a complete list of the medicines, supplements and herbal remedies that the patient is taking.
- **Use of databases:** Specialised software and databases can help identify potential drug interactions.
- **Patient Education:** Patients should be instructed to always inform their carer before taking any new medication or supplement.
- **Regular Monitoring:** Where a drug interaction is possible but necessary, increased monitoring of symptoms or blood levels of the drug may be required.
- **Dose adjustment:** In some cases, the dose of one or both drugs can be adjusted to minimise the risks.

The role of the nurse :

Nurses play a central role in detecting and managing drug interactions. As they are often the first point of contact with the patient, nurses can gather essential information about the medicines being taken and monitor for signs of adverse interactions. In addition, by educating patients about the importance of reporting all the medicines they are taking, the nurse plays a crucial preventive role.

Drug interactions are a constant challenge in the world of medicine, and particularly in psychiatry. Proactive management, combined with sound education and effective communication between carers and patients, can minimise the risks and ensure that treatments are both safe and effective.

Chapter 12:
SPECIAL POPULATIONS
IN PSYCHIATRY

Psychiatry
of children and adolescents.

Child and adolescent psychiatry differs from adult psychiatry in its specific approach to the mental problems of these age groups. Faced with individuals in the throes of physical, emotional and cognitive growth, it requires an in-depth understanding of the phases of development and of family, social and school interactions.

The Peculiarity of Development :
The brain of children and adolescents is constantly evolving. Emotional reactions, behaviours and symptoms can vary according to age and stage of development. An understanding of the normal stages of development is essential to distinguish between what is normal and what may be pathological.

Common Disorders in Children and Adolescents:
- **Autism spectrum disorder:** Affects communication and social behaviour.
- **ADHD (Attention Deficit Disorder with or without Hyperactivity):** Characterised by problems with attention, hyperactivity and impulsivity.
- **Anxiety disorders:** such as phobias, generalised anxiety or obsessive-compulsive disorder.
- **Mood disorders:** such as depression or bipolar disorder.
- Eating disorders: anorexia, bulimia.

- **Psychotic disorders:** Although rarer at this age, they require special attention.

The Impact of Family and Social Context :
The role of the family is central to the lives of children and adolescents. Family dynamics and stressful events such as divorce or moving house can have profound repercussions. Similarly, the school environment, friendships and extra-curricular activities play an essential role in psychological well-being.

Therapeutic management :
- **Individual therapy:** This enables the child or adolescent to express their feelings and work on their problems.
- **Family therapies:** These aim to improve interactions within the family.
- **Group therapies:** Useful for teenagers to share their experiences.
- **Drug treatment:** This may be considered, but always with caution and taking account of specific physiological factors.

The role of the nurse in child psychiatry :
The nurse is often the first point of contact. They assess, observe and play a supportive role. Educating parents and relatives is also essential, enabling a better understanding of the disorders and better management at home.

Child and adolescent psychiatry is a delicate field, which takes into account the complexity of development and social interactions at these ages. Appropriate care, active listening and close collaboration with the family are vital in helping these young patients to navigate the challenges of their lives and lay solid foundations for their future.

Geriatric psychiatry :
Mental disorders in the elderly.

Geriatric psychiatry is a branch of psychiatry dedicated to the management of mental disorders in the elderly. With increasing life expectancy and a growing elderly population, this speciality is becoming more and more relevant and necessary.

Understanding old age :
Old age is accompanied by multiple transformations: physiological, psychological and social. Cognitive changes, physical weakening, gradual loss of autonomy, bereavement, retirement and feelings of isolation can all be sources of stress and vulnerability for the elderly.

Common mental disorders in the elderly :
- **Depressive disorders:** Depression is one of the most common psychiatric pathologies in older people, but it is often under-diagnosed or confused with the manifestations of normal ageing.
- **Neurodegenerative diseases:** such as Alzheimer's or Parkinson's disease. These diseases are often accompanied by psychiatric symptoms, such as mood disorders, hallucinations or delusions.
- **Anxiety disorders:** These can be linked to fear of death, isolation or dependency.
- **Senile psychoses:** Although less common, these require special attention to ensure the safety of the patient and those around them.

Therapeutic management :
- **Full assessment:** This includes a detailed history, physical examination, neuropsychological tests and, if necessary, imaging studies.
- **Non-drug therapies:** such as cognitive-behavioural therapy, music therapy or reminiscence.

- **Drug treatment:** Pharmacology in the elderly is complex due to drug interactions and age-related metabolic changes. Close monitoring is necessary.
- **Support for carers :** The relatives of the elderly play a crucial role. Their support and training can improve the patient's quality of life.

The role of the gerontopsychiatric nurse :
The nurse is at the heart of the care, providing daily monitoring, observing behavioural changes, administering medication and offering psychological support. They work closely with a multidisciplinary team, including the doctor, psychologist and occupational therapist, among others.

Although gerontopsychiatry is a specialised field, it is a reminder of the importance of looking at the whole person. Psychological disorders in the elderly can often be a manifestation of their experiences, concerns or physical suffering. A holistic approach, combining medical expertise with human sensitivity, is therefore essential to offer these individuals the quality of life they deserve.

Psychiatric disorders during pregnancy and post-partum.

Pregnancy and the post-partum period are times of profound physiological, hormonal and psychological upheaval for women. These changes can increase vulnerability to various psychiatric disorders. Recognising and managing these disorders is essential for the well-being of both mother and baby.

Normal Emotional Changes :
It's perfectly normal for women to feel a range of emotions during pregnancy and after giving birth. Mood swings, due to hormonal changes and anxieties about motherhood, can

occur. However, it is crucial to distinguish these normal changes from pathological symptoms.

Common disorders during pregnancy and the post-partum period:
- **Depression:** The "baby blues" are common a few days after childbirth. If this sadness persists or worsens, it could develop into post-partum depression, which requires medical intervention.
- **Post-partum psychosis:** Although rare, it is serious. It can lead to hallucinations, delusions and, in rare cases, dangerous behaviour for the mother or baby.
- **Anxiety disorders:** such as panic disorder, obsessive-compulsive disorder or generalised anxiety disorder, may appear or worsen during this period.
- **Post-childbirth PTSD:** Some women can develop post-traumatic stress disorder following a particularly difficult or traumatic birth.

Risk Factors :
- **Psychiatric history:** Women with a history of psychiatric disorders are at greater risk.
- **Stress and life changes:** Moving house, relationship or financial problems can contribute to the emergence of disorders.
- Complications during pregnancy or childbirth.
- **Lack of support:** A lack of support from a partner, family or friends can exacerbate symptoms.

Therapeutic management :
- **Therapy:** Cognitive-behavioural therapy or interpersonal therapy can be effective.
- **Medication:** Antidepressants can be prescribed, carefully weighing up the benefits and risks for both mother and child.
- **Support:** Support groups can provide a space for sharing and helping each other.

Role of carers :
Early detection is crucial. Doctors, nurses and midwives must be trained to recognise symptoms, offer support and refer to specialists if necessary.

Psychiatric disorders during pregnancy and the post-partum period are serious health problems that can have a lasting impact on the mother, child and family. Awareness, careful monitoring and appropriate management are essential to ensure the long-term well-being of all those involved.

Chapter 13:
CULTURE AND PSYCHIATRY

Influence of culture
on the perception of mental illness.

Culture, a rich tapestry of stories, beliefs and traditions, inevitably influences our perception of the world around us. When it comes to mental health, culture plays a key role, shaping not only how we identify and understand mental illness, but also how we respond to and treat it.

Throughout the ages, in various societies, disorders of the mind have been interpreted in different ways. For some cultures, the symptoms of mental illness could be seen as signs of demonic possession, divine punishment or supernatural gifts. In others, they could be seen as natural imbalances to be rectified by rituals or traditional remedies.

While modernity brings with it advances in science and medicine, these traditional conceptions do not simply disappear. Instead, they often coexist with more medicalised interpretations of mental disorders, creating a complex landscape where cultural beliefs and medical knowledge intersect and sometimes collide.

This confluence can lead to tensions, particularly when mental health professionals, trained in Western settings, interact with patients from diverse cultural backgrounds. A symptom that is considered pathological in one culture may be considered a normal or even valued variation in another. For example, in some cultures, hearing voices may be seen as a spiritual experience rather than a sign of schizophrenia.

In addition, the stigma associated with mental illness varies enormously between cultures. In some contexts, admitting to a struggle with depression or anxiety may result in isolation or discrimination, while in others it may be met with empathy and openness. This cultural variability can influence a person's willingness to seek help or adhere to recommended treatment.

It is therefore essential for mental health professionals to adopt a culturally sensitive approach, recognising that concepts of illness, wellbeing and recovery are not universal, but deeply rooted in the specific cultural contexts of each individual. By understanding and respecting these nuances, they can offer more effective and compassionate care, harmonising modern interventions with the beliefs and values of those they seek to help.

Challenges and strategies for intercultural care.

Intercultural care is a complex and sensitive area of medicine that aims to provide equitable and appropriate healthcare to patients from diverse cultural backgrounds. This approach recognises that culture profoundly influences how individuals perceive health, illness, treatment and care. While the intercultural approach is necessary, it is also fraught with pitfalls and challenges.

Challenges of intercultural care :
- **Language barriers:** Language is the main means of communication between patient and healthcare professional. Lack of mutual understanding can lead to misdiagnosis or poor adherence to treatment.
- **Different beliefs and perceptions:** Beliefs about the cause of illness, preferred treatment methods and

notions of well-being vary considerably from one culture to another.

- **Stigma and discrimination:** In some cultures, particular stigmas are associated with certain illnesses, which can prevent patients from seeking help or sharing their symptoms.
- **Differences in communication standards:** Eye contact, the way questions are asked and receptiveness to information can vary from culture to culture.
- **Institutional constraints:** Healthcare systems are often structured according to Western standards and may not be equipped to manage intercultural nuances.

Strategies for effective intercultural care :
- **Cultural training:** Provide healthcare professionals with training to raise their awareness of different cultural perspectives, health beliefs and health-related behaviours.
- **Interpreting services:** Providing professional interpreters who can facilitate communication between the patient and the healthcare professional.
- **Integrating traditional healers:** In some cultures, traditional healers play an essential role in treatment. Working with them can build trust and improve results.
- **Adopt an attitude of cultural humility:** Rather than assuming complete knowledge of cultures, approach each patient as an opportunity to learn and understand their unique point of view.
- **Appropriate communication methods:** Adapt your communication style to suit the patient's needs and preferences, while paying attention to what is left unsaid and to non-verbal cues.
- **Flexibility in treatment protocols:** Recognise that standard treatments may not be suitable for all

patients and be open to modifying treatment plans according to cultural needs.

- **Creating a welcoming environment:** This could include visual elements representing different cultures or spaces dedicated to prayer and meditation for different religious groups.

Intercultural care is a journey rather than a destination. It requires introspection, ongoing education and a willingness to embrace diversity in all its forms. By overcoming these challenges and adopting these strategies, healthcare professionals can offer truly patient-centred care that respects patients' beliefs, values and cultural identity.

Chapter 14:
THE TECHNOLOGY
AND INNOVATION IN PSYCHIATRY

Telemedicine
and remote consultations.

Telemedicine, which encompasses the use of information and communication technologies to provide medical care at a distance, has revolutionised the world of healthcare. Once seen as a secondary or complementary solution, telemedicine is now recognised as an essential care modality, particularly in situations where access to traditional care is limited or compromised.

Benefits of telemedicine :
* **Accessibility:** It offers care to patients who are geographically distant or have difficulty travelling. This is particularly relevant for rural or underserved areas.
* **Convenience:** Patients can receive care in the comfort of their own home, avoiding travel, waiting times and any associated costs.
* **Continuity   of care:** This enables smooth communication between different care providers, guaranteeing seamless care.
* **Rapid response:** In emergency situations, remote consultations can provide an immediate assessment.
* **Savings:** By reducing the need for physical facilities and travel, telemedicine can lead to savings for providers and patients.

The challenges of telemedicine :
- **Technological limitations:** Not all patients have access to reliable technology or a stable Internet connection.
- **Concerns about confidentiality:** The transmission of medical information via the Internet raises concerns about data protection.
- **Limitations of the physical examination:** Some conditions require a thorough physical examination, which is difficult to carry out remotely.
- **Regulatory issues:** Legislation on telemedicine varies from country to country and can be complicated.

Telemedicine in psychiatry :
In psychiatry, telemedicine has proved particularly useful. Given that psychiatric consultations are largely based on conversations and verbal assessments rather than in-depth physical examinations, they lend themselves well to remote consultations.

- **Initial consultations:** Preliminary psychiatric assessments can be carried out effectively at a distance, enabling rapid evaluation and referral if necessary.
- **Therapy:** Remote therapy, or teletherapy, has become commonplace, enabling patients to continue their treatment despite geographical or logistical obstacles.
- **Medication management:** Psychiatrists can monitor and adjust a patient's medication via remote consultations, although some monitoring may require physical tests.
- **Support groups:** Group therapy sessions can also be organised online, offering community support without the geographical constraints.

Telemedicine in psychiatry, as in other medical fields, requires appropriate training for providers, as well as safeguards to ensure patient confidentiality and safety. However, with the rapid evolution of the technology and growing recognition of its benefits, telemedicine is well on the way to becoming a lasting and valuable part of the medical landscape.

Mobile applications and self-help platforms.

In the digital age, mobile apps and self-help platforms have become an important part of the mental health landscape, offering users a variety of tools to manage, understand and improve their psychological wellbeing.

Advantages of self-help applications and platforms :
- **Availability:** These tools are often available 24 hours a day, offering immediate support when needed.
- **Anonymity:** For those who fear the stigma associated with seeking help for mental health problems, these platforms offer a degree of confidentiality.
- **Cost:** Many applications are free or low-cost, making access to information and support more affordable.
- **Complementarity:** These tools can complement traditional treatment, allowing patients to continue working on themselves between sessions.

Types of applications and platforms :
- **Mood tracking applications:** These tools allow users to track their moods and thoughts on a daily basis, helping to identify triggers or trends.
- **Meditation and mindfulness applications:** These platforms provide guides and meditations to

help reduce stress and anxiety and improve concentration.

- **Therapeutic applications:** These often offer modules based on proven therapies, such as cognitive-behavioural therapy, to manage specific problems.
- **Self-help platforms:** These are often online forums or communities where users can share experiences, ask questions and get support from peers.
- **Therapeutic games:** Some games have been designed to help manage stress, anxiety and other mental health problems.

Important considerations :
- **Reliability:** Not all applications are created equal. It is crucial to choose applications that are based on research and evidence, rather than those that offer quick fixes with no scientific basis.
- **Data security:** Given that these applications deal with sensitive data, it is essential to guarantee the confidentiality and security of the information.
- **Not a substitute:** Although these tools can be invaluable, they should not replace professional therapy, particularly for individuals suffering from serious mental health problems.

With the ever-increasing use of smartphones and mobile devices, self-help applications and platforms are likely to continue to play an increasingly important role in the field of mental health. They offer an innovative and accessible way of providing support to those who need it, while complementing traditional approaches to treatment.

Technological advances in neuroimaging.

Neuroimaging, which encompasses a range of techniques used to visualise the structure and function of the nervous system, has undergone remarkable technological advances in recent decades. These innovations have not only broadened our understanding of the brain, but have also led to significant improvements in the diagnosis, treatment and research of neurological and psychiatric disorders.

1. Magnetic resonance imaging (MRI) :
- **Functional MRI (fMRI)**: This measures and maps brain activity by detecting changes associated with blood flow. It is particularly useful for examining how the brain functions during specific tasks.
- **Diffusion MRI (D-MRI)**: This technique visualises nerve fibre pathways by analysing the movement of water molecules in the brain. It is essential for studying brain connectivity.

2. Positron emission tomography (PET) :
This method uses radioactive tracers to visualise metabolic processes in the brain. It is frequently used to study glucose metabolism in the brain and detect areas of dysfunction.

3. Magnetic resonance spectroscopy :
It analyses specific metabolites in the brain, offering insights into brain chemistry without the need for radioactive products.

4. Magnetoencephalography (MEG) :
This technique detects the tiny magnetic fields produced by neuronal activity. It offers extremely high temporal resolution, making it possible to examine brain activity on millisecond time scales.

5. Optical imaging :
- **Diffuse optical tomography (DOT)**: uses light to obtain detailed images of brain function, particularly useful for imaging the cerebral cortex.
- **Functional near infrared imaging (fNIRS)**: This measures changes in oxygen concentration in the blood to map brain activity.

6. Connectomics :
Based mainly on D-MRI, this emerging discipline aims to map the complex network of connections in the brain, known as the connectome.

Impact of these advances :
- **Disease research**: Advances in neuroimaging have led to the discovery of potential biomarkers for diseases such as Alzheimer's, schizophrenia and depression.
- **Understanding brain connectivity**: We have a better understanding of how different regions of the brain interact and are connected.
- **Image-guided treatment**: In some cases, neuroimaging can guide treatments such as brain surgery.

Technological advances in neuroimaging continue to enrich our understanding of the human brain, offering new perspectives and tools for studying its structure and function, as well as for treating neurological and psychiatric disorders.

Chapter 15:
EMERGING THERAPEUTIC APPROACHES

Therapies based on on mindfulness.

Mindfulness-based therapies are therapeutic approaches that integrate traditional mindfulness meditation practices into a clinical setting. These methods have gained in popularity in recent years, being recognised for their effectiveness in treating a variety of psychological and physical disorders.

Definition of Mindfulness :
Mindfulness is a form of meditation that involves paying benevolent, non-critical and non-reactive attention to present experience, whether it's a sensation, an emotion or a thought.

Main therapies based on mindfulness :
- Mindfulness-based cognitive therapy (MBCT) :
    - Initially designed to prevent relapse in people who have suffered from depression, this therapy combines mindfulness meditation with the principles of cognitive therapy.
    - It teaches how to recognise and defuse the habitual mental patterns that can lead to a relapse into depression.
- Mindfulness-based stress reduction (MBSR) :
    - Developed by Dr. Jon Kabat-Zinn, this approach is often taught in an 8-week course format.
    - It was developed to help people manage stress, pain and illness.

- MBSR is now used for a variety of conditions, including anxiety, depression and chronic pain.
- Acceptance and Commitment Therapy (ACT) :
  - Although not exclusively a mindfulness therapy, ACT incorporates mindfulness concepts to help people accept their internal experience while moving towards actions aligned with their values.

Benefits of mindfulness-based therapies :
- **Stress reduction**: These therapies help to manage and reduce stress by encouraging mindfulness and a calm response to challenges.
- **Emotional regulation**: They teach you to observe your emotions without overreacting or avoiding them.
- **Improved concentration**: Regular meditation practice can improve attention span.
- **Reduction in depressive symptoms**: Especially with MBCT, which is specifically aimed at preventing depressive relapses.
- **Pain management**: Rather than fighting pain, mindfulness teaches us to turn towards sensation with an attitude of acceptance.

Important considerations :
- Although these therapies offer many benefits, they are not a panacea and may not be suitable for everyone. A proper assessment by a professional is always necessary.
- Regular practice is essential to reap all the benefits.

Mindfulness-based therapies offer valuable tools for navigating life's challenges, managing stress, pain and emotions, and can be effectively integrated into a holistic approach to mental and physical well-being.

Virtual reality in psychotherapy.

Virtual reality (VR) has made significant advances in recent years, evolving from a technology largely associated with video games to a tool used in many fields, including psychotherapy. It offers an innovative method of treating a variety of psychological disorders by creating virtual environments where patients can be exposed, interact, learn and adapt.

The use of virtual reality in psychotherapy :
- Virtual Reality Exposure Therapy (VRET):
    - This is the most common use of VR in psychotherapy. In this method, patients are exposed to stimuli or situations that they find anxiety-provoking in a safe virtual environment.
    - This has been shown to be particularly effective in treating specific phobias, such as fear of flying, fear of heights and post-traumatic stress disorder (PTSD).
- Cognitive rehabilitation :
    - Virtual environments are designed to help patients develop or regain cognitive skills, particularly useful for people who have suffered a brain injury or certain forms of dementia.
- Treatment of addiction disorders :
    - VR can be used to expose patients to triggers for their addictions in a controlled setting, allowing them to learn and practise coping strategies.
- Therapy for body image disorders :
    - By using VR, patients can 'see' their bodies in a different way, which can be useful in treating eating disorders and dysmorphophobia.
- Social skills training :
    - For individuals with autism spectrum disorders or social phobia, VR can offer

scenarios for practising social skills in a controlled environment.

Benefits of using VR in psychotherapy :
- **Control and safety**: Therapists can precisely control the virtual environment, guaranteeing patient safety while adapting the therapy to their specific needs.
- **Immersiveness**: The immersive capability of VR allows the patient to feel fully engaged in the environment, which can increase the effectiveness of the therapy.
- **Accessibility**: Situations that would otherwise be difficult or impossible to recreate in the real world can be easily modelled in VR.

Considerations and precautions :
- **Cybersickness**: Some people may experience nausea or dizziness when using VR.
- **Data security**: As with any digital technology, data confidentiality and security must be a priority.
- **Not for everyone**: Although VR offers benefits, it is not necessarily suitable for all patients or all conditions.

Virtual reality opens exciting doors for psychotherapy, offering innovative ways of approaching treatment. As with any intervention, it is essential that therapists are properly trained and carefully assess whether VR is appropriate for each individual patient.

Integrative and holistic approaches.

Integrative and holistic approaches in psychiatry aim to take account of the individual as a whole, not just focusing on symptoms, but seeking to understand and treat the person as a whole: body, mind and social environment.

These approaches have developed as a reaction to more traditional, segmented medicine, and often combine several therapeutic methods, both conventional and alternative.

Understanding the holistic approach :
- Overview :
  - Rather than simply treating a specific symptom, the holistic approach seeks to understand how the different aspects of a person's life interact and contribute to their overall well-being.
- Body-Mind-Environment :
  - Holistic practitioners believe that the body, mind and environment are interdependent. Problems in one of these areas can affect the others, and vice versa.
- Personalised treatment :
  - Each person is unique, with his or her own history, experiences and needs. The holistic approach therefore aims to tailor treatment to the individual, rather than applying a one-size-fits-all solution.

Integrating different therapeutic methods :
- Conventional medicine :
  - Although the approach is holistic, this does not mean that conventional treatments are avoided. On the contrary, they are often used in conjunction with alternative therapies to maximise the benefits for the patient.
- Complementary therapies :
  - These may include acupuncture, chiropractic, naturopathy, reflexology, music therapy, art therapy and many others.

- Traditional medicines :
    - Practices such as Ayurvedic medicine or traditional Chinese medicine can be integrated into a holistic treatment plan.
- Relaxation and stress reduction techniques :
    - Meditation, yoga, tai chi and mindfulness are often recommended to help reduce stress and improve mental health.
- Nutrition :
    - Diet plays an essential role in mental health. A balanced diet, sometimes combined with specific supplements, may be advisable.
- Physical exercise :
    - Physical activity is not only good for the body, but also for the mind. It can help reduce anxiety and depression and improve mood.
- Nature therapy :
    - Contact with nature, whether through walking, gardening or simply contemplation, has been shown to have beneficial effects on mental health.

Considerations and challenges :
- Cultural resistance :
    - In certain cultures or environments, the holistic approach may be viewed with scepticism, especially if it is seen as being far removed from 'traditional' medicine.
- Search for :
    - While some complementary therapies have been well studied, others lack robust research to confirm their effectiveness.
- Cost :
    - Some holistic treatments or therapies may not be covered by health insurance, making access difficult for all patients.

The integrative and holistic approach to psychiatry recognises that mental health is complex and multifactorial. By embracing a variety of therapeutic methods and tailoring them to the individual, this approach aims to promote lasting recovery and overall well-being.

Chapter 16:
RESEARCH IN PSYCHIATRY AND FUTURE PROSPECTS

Importance of research clinical and fundamental.

Research, whether clinical or fundamental, is the driving force behind all medical advances. In the field of psychiatry, it is a compass that guides professionals towards a better understanding of mental disorders and ever more effective treatments.

Fundamental research, often carried out in the laboratory, explores the mysteries of the brain, a complex organ which, despite technological advances, remains largely unknown. It is through this research that we discover the biochemical, genetic and cellular mechanisms underlying psychiatric disorders. These discoveries, sometimes unexpected, are essential because they lay the foundations for new hypotheses, new treatments and new therapeutic approaches.

On the other hand, clinical research is closely linked to day-to-day practice in psychiatry. It involves studying patients themselves, often in the form of clinical trials. It is through clinical research that we can assess the efficacy and safety of new treatments, or gain a better understanding of the natural course of disorders. Among other things, it makes it possible to adapt and optimise therapeutic approaches according to the specific needs of each patient.

The interaction between these two types of research is vital. Discoveries made in basic research can inspire new therapies, which can then be tested in the clinic. Conversely, clinical observations can raise new questions for basic research.

But psychiatric research is more than just a medical advance; it also has a societal role to play. By demystifying mental illness, it helps to combat the stigma associated with it. By shedding light on the underlying biological mechanisms, it reminds us that psychiatric disorders are illnesses like any others, deserving of attention, care and respect.

Finally, research is also a beacon of hope. Every discovery, every new clinical trial is a promise for patients and their families: the promise that, tomorrow, we will have more effective tools, more appropriate treatments, and that we will be able to offer a better quality of life to those affected by psychiatric disorders.

In short, research, both clinical and fundamental, is at the heart of modern psychiatry. It is shaping the future of the discipline and guaranteeing ever more precise, individualised and humane care.

The latest key discoveries.

Advances in psychiatry, as in many other areas of medicine, are the result of relentless research efforts. These scientific advances, which are regularly updated, are essential for refining our knowledge, improving patient care and renewing our therapeutic approaches. Here is an overview of some of the most significant discoveries in psychiatry in recent years:

- **The intestinal microbiota and mental health**: Research has revealed a link between the intestinal microbiota (all the micro-organisms present in our intestines) and our brain, dubbed the "intestine-brain axis". Studies have shown that an imbalance in this microbiota could be associated with various mental disorders, including depression.
- **Advanced neuroimaging**: Thanks to imaging technologies such as functional MRI, we are now able to observe brain activity in real time. This has led to a better understanding of the patterns of activity associated with certain disorders and the identification of potential biomarkers.
- **Gene therapies and epigenetics**: By identifying specific genes linked to certain psychiatric disorders, researchers are exploring approaches to target these genes via gene therapies or to understand how the environment can influence gene expression through epigenetics.
- **Integrative approach to autism spectrum disorders (ASD)**: The understanding of ASD has been greatly enhanced by genetic, neurological and behavioural studies. This has led to more targeted and personalised interventions for affected individuals.
- **The use of psychedelics in psychotherapy**: Substances such as psilocybin, found in certain varieties of mushrooms, are being studied for their potential therapeutic applications, particularly in the treatment of resistant depression.
- **Deep brain stimulation (DBS)**: DBS, which involves implanting small electrodes in the brain, has shown promising results in the treatment of disorders such as resistant major depression and obsessive-compulsive disorder.
- **The importance of sleep**: Research has reinforced the idea that sleep plays a crucial role in mental

health. Disorders such as depression, anxiety and psychosis can be exacerbated or even triggered by a chronic lack of sleep.

These discoveries, among many others, demonstrate the richness and dynamism of research in psychiatry. They reinforce the hope that, in the future, we will have even more effective means of diagnosing, treating and, ideally, preventing mental illness.

Future prospects and therapeutic innovations.

Psychiatry, like the medical field as a whole, is at a crossroads of exciting innovations that promise to radically transform our understanding and treatment of mental illness. The outlook for the future is marked not only by technological advances, but also by an increasingly holistic and patient-centred approach. Here are some of the most promising trends and therapeutic innovations to watch out for:

- **Personalised medicine**: In the future, psychiatric treatments will be increasingly personalised, based on the genetics, metabolism and individual characteristics of each patient. This will make it possible to optimise interventions to obtain the best possible results.
- **Digital therapies**: Increasingly, therapies based on mobile applications or online platforms will be integrated into treatment plans. They can offer real-time support, help manage symptoms or act as self-monitoring tools.
- **Neurofeedback and biofeedback**: These techniques enable patients to become aware of and regulate their physiological functions. For example, by

viewing their brain activity in real time, patients can learn to modulate certain patterns of activity associated with their symptoms.

- **Increased use of virtual reality (VR)**: VR can be used to treat disorders such as PTSD, by gradually exposing patients to triggering stimuli in a controlled environment.

- **The expansion of psychedelic therapies**: As mentioned above, substances such as psilocybin and MDMA are being studied for their potential therapeutic properties, particularly for depression, anxiety and PTSD.

- **Non-invasive brain stimulation**: Techniques such as transcranial magnetic stimulation (TMS) can offer an alternative to drugs for certain patients, by modulating brain activity without surgery.

- **Community-centred approaches**: Rather than focusing solely on the individual, there is a growing recognition of the importance of community support. Care will increasingly be rooted in a systemic approach, integrating family, educators and social workers.

- **Increased emphasis on prevention**: Rather than treating symptoms alone, there will be a growing effort to identify and treat risk factors before they lead to more serious disorders.

- **Integration of mental and physical health**: Recognising that the mind and body are inextricably linked, there will be a growing fusion of psychiatric and somatic care to provide a more holistic approach to health.

- **Increased training and awareness**: As the stigma surrounding mental illness decreases, there will be an increased demand for education, training and awareness-raising, both for healthcare professionals and the general public.

The future of psychiatry looks bright, marked by a better understanding of mental disorders and increasingly effective treatments tailored to individual needs.

Chapter 17:
FORENSIC PSYCHIATRY

The intersection of psychiatry and the judicial system.

The intersection of psychiatry and the justice system is a complex area where medicine, ethics and the law meet. It raises crucial questions about individual rights, the protection of society and the role of mental health professionals within the justice system. Let us approach this subject in a fluid and integrated way.

History and background
Historically, the understanding of mental illness has often been biased and misinformed, leading to prejudice and stigmatisation. Individuals with mental disorders were once perceived as possessed or morally defective, leading to their isolation or inappropriate punishment. With the progress of science and a better understanding of psychiatry, society has gradually recognised the importance of treating mental illness as a medical rather than a criminal issue.

Criminal Liability and Mental Capacity
A central question at this intersection is that of criminal responsibility. Can a person suffering from a serious mental illness be held responsible for his or her criminal acts? In many jurisdictions, an insanity defence or 'insanity defence' may be invoked, recognising that an individual may lack the capacity to understand the nature of his or her actions or to discern right from wrong.

Forensic Psychiatric Assessment

When an individual is suspected of suffering from a mental illness, psychiatric assessments may be requested to determine his or her capacity to appear in court. These assessments may also help to inform the court about the need for specific treatments or interventions.

Psychiatric hospitals and detention centres
In some cases, individuals with serious mental illness who have committed crimes are not incarcerated in traditional prisons, but are instead placed in specialised psychiatric institutions for treatment.

Ethical issues

The intersection of psychiatry and the justice system raises important ethical questions. For example, how far can society go in forcing a person to undergo psychiatric treatment? What rights do individuals who are involuntarily hospitalised have?

Rehabilitation and reintegration

Another crucial aspect is rehabilitation. How can the justice system and mental health professionals work together to ensure that individuals, once released, reintegrate safely and effectively into society?

L'Avenir

As the understanding of mental illness continues to evolve, the intersection of psychiatry and the justice system will require constant reflection and adjustment to ensure that the rights of individuals are respected while protecting society as a whole.

Ultimately, the balance between justice and compassion, between security and human rights, remains a constant challenge in this interdisciplinary field.

Assessment of dangerousness and criminal liability.

Psychiatry plays a major role in addressing the question of an individual's dangerousness and criminal responsibility. Let's decipher this complex issue by combining law and medicine.

Origins and background
Assessing dangerousness has always been a key element of criminal justice. Over time, society has sought to introduce objective, evidence-based assessments to determine the likelihood of an individual committing a violent or harmful act in the future.

Assessment mechanisms
The first stage of the assessment is usually a thorough psychiatric examination. Health professionals assess the individual's history, current thinking and behaviour, as well as any underlying factors that may increase the risk of violent acts, such as untreated mental illness.

Mental illness vs. criminal liability
One of the central questions in this assessment is whether a mental illness has directly contributed to criminal behaviour. A distinction is made between an individual's ability to understand their actions and to distinguish right from wrong. If an individual is deemed incapable of this understanding because of a mental illness, he or she may be considered not criminally responsible.

Future danger
A crucial part of the assessment is determining the risk of re-offending. Although predicting future behaviour is complex, certain methods, such as actuarial assessments, are used to estimate risk based on demographic factors, criminal history and other relevant variables.

If an individual is judged to be dangerous but not responsible for their actions due to mental illness, they can be placed in a psychiatric hospital for an indefinite period. This placement may last longer than the traditional prison sentence they would have received.

Ethical issues
The tension between public safety and individual rights is clear. On the one hand, it is essential to protect society from potentially dangerous individuals. On the other, it is imperative to ensure that individuals receive fair and ethical treatment, particularly when mental illness is at stake.

Assessing dangerousness and criminal responsibility is a delicate process that requires close collaboration between the judicial system and mental health professionals. In seeking a balance between compassion, justice and public safety, it remains essential to approach each case with rigour, ethics and humanity.

Patient management in prisons.

The intersection between psychiatry and the prison environment is a complex terrain, requiring careful attention to both the safety of the prisoner and their mental health needs. Let's explore this delicate relationship and the best practices for managing patients in prison.

The Face of Mental Health in Prison
Alarmingly, many inmates in prisons around the world show symptoms of mental disorders. These disorders can range from mild depression to more serious conditions such as schizophrenia. There are a number of reasons for this, ranging from the criminalisation of mental illness to the lack of adequate care systems in society.

Initial Assessment

As soon as a prisoner arrives, an initial psychiatric assessment is crucial. This enables existing disorders to be detected, the risk of suicide or self-aggression to be assessed, and the detainee to be directed towards appropriate treatment.

Carceral Environment and Risks

Prison can aggravate the symptoms of mental disorders. Isolation, the stress of prison life, victimisation and other factors can contribute to the deterioration of an inmate's mental health. Hence the importance of regular monitoring.

Therapeutic Interventions

Interventions in prisons can include pharmacotherapy, individual or group therapy, and educational programmes. However, the challenge often lies in implementing these interventions in a constrained and secure environment.

The Question of Isolation

Isolation or solitary confinement is a controversial practice, particularly for mentally ill prisoners. Although sometimes used for disciplinary reasons, this method can have devastating consequences for mental health.

Social reintegration

Preparing prisoners for their release is as crucial as looking after their mental health while they are in prison. This involves coordination with mental health and social services on the outside, to ensure a smooth transition and continuation of treatment.

Ethical Challenges

Healthcare professionals working in prisons are often caught between their duty to care for prisoners and the security requirements of the prison administration. This tension can give rise to major ethical dilemmas.

Managing mental health in prisons is a multidimensional task that requires a balanced approach, taking into account the safety, ethics and well-being of the prisoner. By recognising and responding to the needs of this vulnerable population, society can hope to reduce recidivism and promote successful reintegration.

Chapter 18:
THE NURSE TRAINER AND LEADER

Sharing knowledge
with the new nurses.

The arrival of a new nurse on a psychiatric ward is both a challenge and an opportunity. It's an opportunity for experienced nurses to pass on their knowledge, tips and values. Sharing knowledge not only enhances the efficiency of the nursing team, it also ensures continuity of quality care for patients.

A Living Memory
Over the years, each nurse becomes a living memory of his or her department. They remember patients, complex cases, successes and failures. This wealth of experience is invaluable to a newcomer, who often feels a little lost in this new environment.

Structured Transmission
It's not just about telling anecdotes. The transmission of knowledge must be structured. This can take the form of in-house training sessions, debriefings after complex situations or supervision time.

The Art of Communication
Passing on knowledge also means knowing how to communicate. It means putting yourself in the new nurse's shoes, understanding their concerns and questions. It also means knowing how to listen, because new nurses can also bring a fresh perspective and recently acquired knowledge.

Sharing Tools
With today's technology, knowledge-sharing tools abound. Whether it's online platforms, internal forums or videoconferencing sessions, it's become easier to share and communicate, even from a distance.

The Importance of Kindness
In this sharing of knowledge, it is crucial to maintain a benevolent attitude. To err is human, and new nurses need to feel confident to ask questions, admit their shortcomings and learn from their mistakes.

Mentoring
Some departments set up mentoring systems, where an experienced nurse is assigned to a newcomer to guide them through their first steps. This is an excellent way of ensuring a smooth transition and optimal learning.

Sharing your knowledge with new nurses is not just a professional duty, it's an asset. It's the assurance of a close-knit, competent team ready to face the challenges of psychiatry with empathy and expertise.

Coaching, supervision and mentoring.

At the heart of any medical profession, the continuity and quality of care depend to a large extent on the ability of experienced practitioners to pass on their knowledge and guide those who are less experienced. Coaching, supervision and mentoring play essential roles in this transmission. Each of these terms contains specific nuances and functions that help to ensure not only clinical competence, but also the well-being and professional development of carers.

1. Management: Structure and Support

Coaching refers to the establishment of structures and processes to guide nurses, especially younger nurses, in their daily practice. These include:

- **Initial training**: Introducing new nurses to the establishment's protocols and policies.
- **Evaluation**: Provide regular feedback on performance and identify areas for improvement.
- **Day-to-day support**: Helping nurses to manage challenges and difficult situations.

2. Supervision: a deepening of know-how

Supervision is a more intimate and regular process, focused on the professional and personal development of nurses. It involves:

- **Reflection on practice**: Analysing complex situations and discussing ethical dilemmas.
- **Skills development**: Identifying gaps in knowledge or skills and working to improve them.
- **Emotional Support**: Providing a space to talk about the stresses and emotional challenges of the profession.

3. Mentoring: A Coaching Relationship

Mentoring is a professional relationship in which a more experienced nurse (the mentor) offers advice, support and guidance to a less experienced nurse (the mentee). This relationship may include:

- **Passing on knowledge**: sharing experience and tips acquired over time.
- **Professional Support**: Helping the mentee navigate their career, identify opportunities and make decisions.
- **Personal Development**: Encouraging personal growth, self-confidence and resilience.

Coaching, supervision and mentoring are three essential pillars for ensuring continuous, high-quality training in the field of psychiatry. These approaches structure nurses' professional development, strengthen team cohesion and guarantee better patient care.

The nurse as leader and changemaker.

Over the years, the nursing profession has evolved considerably, moving from a passive role of execution to a proactive role of leadership in the medical field. Today, nurses are not only care providers, but also agents of change, opinion leaders, researchers and patient advocates.

1. The Nurse: A Leader in Medical Teams
Nurses have in-depth knowledge of patients' needs. This expertise makes them natural leaders in medical teams. They coordinate care, facilitate communication between the various professionals and ensure that each patient receives the right treatment.

2. The Role of Nurses in Training and Education
Many nurses are involved in training their colleagues, whether through mentoring, formal courses or information sessions. They share their knowledge and experience to improve the quality of care and enhance the skills of their teams.

3. The nurse as Patients' Rights Defender
Nurses often act as patient advocates, ensuring that patients' rights are respected and that their voices are heard. They may be involved in discussions about medical decisions or national health policies.

4. Participation in Clinical Research

More and more nurses are involved in clinical research, bringing their unique perspective and contributing to the development of care practices.

5. The Changemaker: Leading Change in the Health Sector

Nurses are often at the forefront of initiatives to improve healthcare systems. Whether through technological innovations, new methods of care or awareness campaigns, they lead change, ensuring that it benefits patients.

Nurses, with their proximity to patients and in-depth knowledge of the healthcare system, are ideally placed to be leaders and agents of change. By adopting a proactive approach, continually training themselves and collaborating with other professionals, nurses can truly transform the healthcare landscape and improve the quality of care for all. This role of leader and changemaker is essential if we are to meet the current and future challenges facing the medical sector.

Chapter 19:
CHALLENGES AND TABOOS PSYCHIATRY

Demystifying stereotypes and prejudices surrounding mental illness.

Mental illness, despite the considerable progress made in understanding its mechanisms and in raising public awareness, is still subject to many prejudices. These stereotypes can have devastating consequences, both for people with mental disorders and for society as a whole.

1. The Nature of Stereotypes
Stereotypes are simplified and generalised beliefs about a group of people. In the context of mental illness, these stereotypes can take various forms, such as:
*   People with mental illness are dangerous and unpredictable.
*   These illnesses are the result of a weakness of character or a moral failing.
*   Individuals can simply 'get away with it' if they wish.

2. The Origins of Prejudice
Prejudice against mental disorders has a variety of origins:
*   **History and culture**: In many cultures, mental illness has been associated with supernatural causes or has been perceived as divine punishment.
*   **Media**: Media representations can often exaggerate or misrepresent mental illness, reinforcing stereotypes.

- **Lack of education**: Simple ignorance or misunderstanding of the facts can lead to incorrect judgements.

3. Consequences of stereotypes
Prejudice and stereotypes can have serious consequences:
- **Stigmatisation**: Sufferers may be ostracised, marginalised or shunned by their community.
- **Avoiding care**: For fear of being judged, some people may avoid seeking help or talking about their problems.
- **Discrimination**: At work, at school or in other spheres of life, individuals may face direct or indirect discrimination.

4. Countering stereotypes
It is imperative to combat these prejudices:
- **Education**: Informing the general public about the real nature of mental disorders and demystifying misconceptions.
- **Testimonials**: Encouraging those affected to share their experiences in order to humanise and personalise mental illness.
- **Media responsibility**: Encourage a fair and balanced portrayal of mental illness in the media.
- **Raising awareness**: Organise campaigns, workshops and seminars to raise public awareness.

Mental illness, like any medical condition, requires understanding, compassion and support. By educating society and combating prejudice, we can help to create an environment where individuals are judged on their character and actions, not on stereotypes and misunderstandings.

The importance of fighting against stigmatisation.

From time immemorial, stigma has been a companion of mental illness. It refers to the idea that those affected are somehow inferior, weak or dangerous. Combating this stigma is not only a question of social justice, it is also essential for the well-being and recovery of the individuals concerned.

1. The devastating effects of stigma
Stigma can have a dramatic impact on people's lives:
- **Self-stigmatisation**: The people concerned may internalise these negative attitudes, which damages their self-esteem.
- **Social isolation**: Fearing judgement, sufferers may isolate themselves, exacerbating their condition.
- **Discrimination at work**: Professional opportunities can be reduced, not because of competence, but because of prejudice.
- **Reluctance to seek help**: Stigma can prevent people from seeking treatment, prolonging and exacerbating their suffering.
-

2. Crucial Education
Most stereotypes stem from a lack of understanding:
- **Awareness-raising**: Educational programmes in schools and communities to provide accurate and up-to-date information on mental illness.
- **Personal accounts**: Letting those affected share their experiences can demystify mental illness.

3. The Media: A Double Edge
The media play an essential role in shaping public opinion:
- **Responsibility**: The media should avoid perpetuating harmful stereotypes and seek to educate rather than sensationalise.

- **Highlighting success stories**: highlighting the stories of people who manage their mental illness effectively, showing that they can lead fulfilling lives.

4. The Role of the Medical Community
Mental health professionals must also play their part:
- **Holistic approach**: treating the patient as a whole, not just his or her illness.
- **Open communication**: Encourage patients to ask questions and express their concerns to dispel fears.

5. Involving the Community
It's a collective effort:
- **Community programmes**: Encourage initiatives that promote inclusion and understanding.
- **Open dialogue**: Encourage forums where people can discuss mental health openly without fear of judgement.

Combating stigma is a fundamental step towards enabling everyone to live in a society where mental illness is understood and not feared. Every step towards eradicating stigma is a step towards a more inclusive, caring and healthy society.

Contemporary challenges
the profession of psychiatric nurse.

At the intersection of medical science, human relations and societal developments, the profession of psychiatric nursing faces complex and varied challenges. As the field of psychiatry undergoes rapid change, new challenges emerge, requiring resilient, well-trained nurses capable of adapting.

1. The ongoing destigmatisation of mental illness
Despite progress, the stigma associated with mental disorders persists, influencing not only public perception but also that of patients themselves.

2. Rapidly evolving treatments
- **New therapies**: Nurses need to keep constantly abreast of therapeutic advances, whether in the form of new medications or alternative therapies.
- **Digital therapies**: The boom in telemedicine and mental wellness applications requires a familiarity with technology.

3. Lack of resources
Many institutions suffer from a chronic lack of resources, whether in terms of staff, funding or equipment.

4. Cultural and Social Complexities
Care must be adapted to the different cultural, social and individual realities of patients. The rise of gender, identity and ethnic diversity issues introduces additional nuances into care.

5. The risks of burnout
The emotionally intense nature of psychiatric work, combined with sometimes long working hours, can lead to burnout and even mental health problems among the carers themselves.

6. Navigation between Autonomy and Safety
Assessing when to prioritise patient autonomy and when to introduce safety measures can be a delicate balancing act.

7. Interprofessional collaboration
Working in synergy with other health professionals (psychiatrists, psychologists, social workers) requires communication and collaboration skills, in an environment that is sometimes fraught with tension.

8. Ethical dilemmas
Issues of confidentiality, informed consent and forced care, for example, can pose delicate ethical dilemmas.

9. Continuing education
The need for ongoing training to keep up to date in a constantly evolving field, while managing day-to-day responsibilities, can be a challenge in itself.

10. Crisis Management
Emergency situations, whether involving suicide attempts, aggression or other crises, require special skills, training and resilience.

Psychiatric nurses are witnessing first-hand the rapid changes taking place in the field of mental health. They play an essential role in patient care, but must also navigate through a sea of challenges that test their skills, patience and resilience. Recognising and addressing these challenges is crucial to ensuring quality care, but also to the well-being of nurses themselves.

Chapter 20:
WELL-BEING AND
THE RESILIENCE OF THE NURSE

Recognise
and manage work-related stress.

Occupational stress is a pervasive issue for many professionals, particularly those working in the healthcare sector. Psychiatric nurses, faced with the heavy responsibilities and emotionally-charged nature of their profession, are particularly exposed. Knowing how to recognise it and deal with it is essential for career continuity, personal well-being and, above all, ensuring quality care for patients.

1. Understanding Occupational Stress
   - **Definition**: A state of physical, emotional or mental tension resulting from stressful factors at work.
   - **Specific causes in psychiatry**: emergency situations, emotional confrontations, ethical dilemmas, time pressures, emotional exhaustion, among others.

2. Recognising Symptoms
   - **Physical**: Fatigue, headaches, sleep problems, muscle tension, digestive problems.
   - **Emotional**: Irritability, anxiety, depression, feelings of exhaustion, reduced self-esteem.
   - **Mental**: Difficulty concentrating, obsessive thoughts, pessimism, social isolation.
   - **Behavioural**: Procrastination, absence from work, increased alcohol or substance abuse.

3. Identifying risk factors
- **External**: High workload, lack of resources, interpersonal conflicts, lack of recognition.
- **Internal**: Perfectionism, lack of time management or communication skills, difficulty setting limits.

4. Prevention and management strategies
- **Self-evaluation**: Take the time to reflect regularly on your emotional and physical state.
- **Continuing training**: Acquire additional skills to better manage professional challenges.
- **Time management**: prioritise tasks, learn to delegate, take regular breaks.
- **Setting limits**: Knowing how to say no, recognising your own limits and taking days off.
- **Support network**: Cultivate relationships with colleagues, friends or a mental health professional to share concerns.
- **Relaxing activities**: Meditation, yoga, reading, or any other activity that relaxes and takes your mind off work pressures.
- **Take care of your health**: eat a balanced diet, exercise regularly and get enough sleep.

5. The Importance of Asking for Help
- **Recognise your own limits**: Admitting that you may need help is not a sign of weakness, but of wisdom.
- **Consult a professional**: A psychologist, psychiatrist or guidance counsellor can offer valuable insights and tools.

Faced with the many challenges of the profession, the recognition and management of professional stress must be at the heart of psychiatric nurses' concerns. It's an essential part of ensuring quality care and preserving mental health. Knowing yourself, equipping yourself with the right tools and not hesitating to seek help are the keys to effectively managing stress at work.

The importance of supervision and continuing education.

The dynamic and complex nature of psychiatry requires nurses to constantly develop their knowledge and skills. In this context, supervision and continuing education are essential pillars in guaranteeing optimal patient care and supporting nurses' well-being and professional development.

1. Supervision: A Reflective Mirror
- **Professional reflection**: Supervision provides a privileged space where nurses can analyse and discuss their practices, their feelings and their questions.
- **Personal growth**: Confronted with situations that can sometimes be destabilising, supervision provides nurses with a place to express their emotions and benefit from benevolent and constructive feedback.
- **Managing ethical dilemmas**: Psychiatry, with its nuances and complexities, often presents ethically ambiguous cases. Supervision helps to clarify and navigate these grey areas.

2. Continuing Education: A Commitment to Excellence
- **Keeping up to date**: Psychiatric research is constantly evolving. Continuing education enables us to keep abreast of the latest discoveries and recommendations.
- **Acquiring new skills**: Patients' needs change, as do therapeutic approaches. Continuous training ensures that we can respond optimally to these needs.

- **Responding to contemporary challenges**: Faced with the emergence of new problems (addictions to new technologies, disorders linked to social upheaval), training enables us to provide appropriate responses.

3. Collateral Benefits
   - **Boosting self-confidence**: Feeling up-to-date and supervised reinforces your sense of competence and professional effectiveness.
   - **Professional networking**: Training courses and supervision sessions provide opportunities to meet and exchange ideas with other professionals in the field, thereby enriching your practice.
   - **Preventing burnout**: By providing a forum for discussion and learning, supervision and ongoing training play a protective role against burnout.

4. Institutional and personal commitment
   - **Institutional responsibility**: It is essential that institutions recognise the importance of supervision and training, allocating time and resources for these purposes.
   - **Individual proactivity**: Each nurse, aware of the value of these tools, should actively seek to benefit from and invest in training and supervision opportunities.

Supervision and continuing education are not simply supplements to the psychiatric nurse's day-to-day work, but absolute necessities. They guarantee the quality of care, nurture professional growth and support psychological well-being. In a field as demanding and changing as psychiatry, stopping to learn is not an option, it's a responsibility.

Taking care of yourself
to take better care of others.

The profession of psychiatric nursing is intrinsically demanding, oscillating between moments of emotional intensity and moments of pure therapeutic bliss. Yet part of the key to effective, empathetic patient care lies in the nurse's ability to take care of themselves. This self-preservation is not a selfish act, but a necessity to ensure optimal quality of care.

1. The Interconnection of Being
   - **Emotional reciprocity**: Nurses, by virtue of their role, are receptacles for their patients' emotions. If not managed properly, these emotions can affect their own mental health.
   - **The mirror of well-being**: Nurses who are happy, serene and at ease with themselves are more likely to inspire confidence and peace of mind in their patients.

2. Self-care techniques and practices
   - **Meditation and mindfulness**: These practices help you to focus, reduce stress and gain perspective on events.
   - **Physical activity**: Exercise, whether gentle like yoga or more intense like running, is a valuable outlet for the body and mind.
   - **Hobbies and passions**: Devoting yourself to extra-professional activities helps you to decompress and reconnect with yourself.
   - **Therapeutic consultations**: Psychotherapy or coaching sessions can help you to discuss your feelings and find coping strategies.

3. The Importance of Borders
   - **Work-personal boundaries**: It is crucial to establish a clear boundary between professional and personal life, to prevent the risk of burnout or over-investment.
   - **Saying no**: Sometimes you have to say no to certain tasks or requests in order to preserve your physical and emotional integrity.

4. Recognition and acceptance
   - **Accepting your limits**: Acknowledging your weaknesses or moments of fatigue is not a defeat, but a necessary realisation to recharge your batteries.
   - **Celebrate small victories**: Congratulating yourself on your daily successes boosts your self-esteem and motivation.

By looking after themselves and cultivating their well-being, psychiatric nurses indirectly offer their patients a healthier, more harmonious therapeutic environment. Taking care of yourself is not a luxury; it's a responsibility towards yourself and towards those you help on a daily basis. Ultimately, a well-balanced nurse is a valuable asset in the world of psychiatry.

CONCLUSION

The future of psychiatry and psychiatric nursing.

Over the years, psychiatry has evolved in parallel with technological, scientific and societal advances. Today, the field is at a major turning point, permeated by medical discoveries, the integration of technology and a renewed emphasis on holistic patient care. The role of the psychiatric nurse is also changing, adapting traditional methods to contemporary needs.

1. More personalised medicine
   - **Precision psychiatry**: The ability to target treatments according to each individual's genetic and biochemical profile could lead to more appropriate and effective care.
   - **Integrative approaches**: The integration of different disciplines, such as nutrition, physiotherapy or art therapy, to provide a comprehensive approach.

2. Integration of Advanced Technologies
   - **Digital therapies**: The use of self-help applications and platforms is likely to become more common.
   - **Virtual reality**: This technology could be used to treat disorders such as phobia or PTSD.
   - **Artificial intelligence**: for diagnostic assistance, patient monitoring and treatment optimisation.

3. Changes in Training and Practice
   - **Ongoing training**: Nurses will need to continually update their skills to stay at the cutting edge of innovative practices.

- **Expanded role for nurses**: With a more patient-centred approach, nurses will be able to play an even more central role in the coordination and delivery of care.

4. A more human approach
- **Combating stigma**: Greater public awareness and education about mental disorders.
- **Focus on prevention**: Early identification of signs and symptoms, with faster intervention.

5. Multi-disciplinary collaboration
- **Teamwork**: Greater coordination between psychiatrists, nurses, social workers and other health professionals to ensure comprehensive care.
- **Holistic care centres**: Facilities offering a full range of services, from diagnosis to rehabilitation.

The future of psychiatry and psychiatric nursing looks promising, with a multitude of opportunities for improvement and innovation. This evolution, while remaining patient-centred, will strive to provide high quality, responsive and integrative care, reflecting the changing needs of society. The fusion of technology, science and humanism paves the way for a future in which psychiatric care is both effective and deeply empathetic.

Encouraging research and innovation.

Psychiatry, like other medical fields, is constantly evolving. It is shaped by scientific discoveries, new therapeutic approaches and the changing needs of patients and society. However, if it is to continue to progress, it is essential to promote research and innovation. These two elements, working in synergy, are the driving force behind improvements in patient care and well-being.

1. The Foundations of the Importance of Research
Clinical and basic research is crucial to our understanding of mental disorders, from their causes to their treatment. It is thanks to this research that we now have more effective medicines, validated psychotherapeutic interventions and preventive strategies.

2. Pushing back the frontiers of knowledge
Innovation in psychiatry is not limited to pharmacology. It encompasses fields as varied as neuroimaging, neuromodulation, gene therapy and artificial intelligence. These innovations have the potential to revolutionise the way we understand, diagnose and treat mental disorders.

3. Create a Favourable Environment
- **Institutional support**: Universities, hospitals and other institutions must recognise the importance of psychiatric research and allocate sufficient resources.
- **Funding**: Governments, private organisations and public-private partnerships must invest in psychiatric research and innovation.
- **Collaborative networks**: Encouraging collaboration between researchers, clinicians, patients and other healthcare professionals to cross-fertilise expertise and perspectives.

4. Educating for innovation
It is essential to incorporate the importance of research and innovation into the training of nurses and other healthcare professionals. They must be encouraged to ask questions, to challenge established methods and to constantly seek improvements.

5. Innovation at the service of patients
At the heart of all these efforts is the patient. Every discovery, every innovation is aimed at improving their quality of life, reducing suffering and restoring mental health. It is by remembering this ultimate goal that psychiatric research and innovation will continue to flourish.

Encouraging research and innovation in psychiatry is not only necessary, it is vital. At a time when mental disorders are becoming increasingly complex, and in the face of societal and environmental challenges, it is more urgent than ever to promote a psychiatry that is enlightened, progressive and resolutely forward-looking.

www.ingramcontent.com/pod-product-compliance
Lightning Source LLC
Chambersburg PA
CBHW062318290526
45794CB00005B/1829